HEALTHCARE IN MOTION

WORLDS IN MOTION

Edited by Noel B. Salazar, University of Leuven, in collaboration with ANTHROMOB, the EASA Anthropology and Mobility Network.

This transdisciplinary series features empirically grounded studies that disentangle how people, objects, and ideas move across the planet. With a special focus on advancing theory as well as methodology, the series considers movement as both an object and a method of study.

Volume 1
KEYWORDS OF MOBILITY
Critical Engagements
Edited by Noel B. Salazar and Kiran Jayaram

Volume 2
METHODOLOGIES OF MOBILITY
Ethnography and Experiment
Edited by Roger Norum, Alice Elliot, and Noel B. Salazar

Volume 3
INTIMATE MOBILITIES
Sexual Economies, Marriage and Migration in a Disparate World
Edited by Christian Groes and Nadine T. Fernandez

Volume 4
MOMENTOUS MOBILITIES
Anthropological Musings on the Meanings of Travel
Noel B. Salazar

Volume 5
HEALTHCARE IN MOTION
Immobilities in Health Service Delivery and Access
Edited by Cecilia Vindrola-Padros, Ginger A. Johnson, and Anne E. Pfister

Healthcare in Motion

Immobilities in Health Service Delivery and Access

Edited by

Cecilia Vindrola-Padros, Ginger A. Johnson, and Anne E. Pfister

berghahn
NEW YORK • OXFORD
www.berghahnbooks.com

First published in 2018 by
Berghahn Books
www.berghahnbooks.com

Library of Congress Cataloging-in-Publication Data

Names: Vindrola-Padros, Cecilia, 1983– editor.
Title: Healthcare in motion : immobilities in health service delivery and access / edited by Cecilia Vindrola-Padros, Ginger A. Johnson, and Anne E. Pfister.
Description: New York : Berghahn Books, 2018. | Series: Worlds in motion ; volume 5 | Includes bibliographical references and index.
Identifiers: LCCN 2018006185 (print) | LCCN 2018018667 (ebook) | ISBN 9781785339547 (ebook) | ISBN 9781785339530 (hardback : alk. paper)
Subjects: LCSH: Health services accessibility. | Health planning. | Medical policy—Social aspects. | Minorities—Medical care.
Classification: LCC RA393 (ebook) | LCC RA393 .H3746 2018 (print) | DDC 362.1—dc23
LC record available at https://lccn.loc.gov/2018006185

British Library Cataloguing in Publication Data

A catalogue record for this book is available from the British Library

ISBN 978-1-78533-953-0 hardback
ISBN 978-1-78533-954-7 ebook

Contents

List of Figures and Tables vii

Introduction Healthcare in Motion 1
Cecilia Vindrola-Padros, Ginger A. Johnson, and Anne E. Pfister

Part I. Healthcare and Differential Mobility Empowerments 15
Cecilia Vindrola-Padros

Chapter 1 "Stuck in Motion": Simultaneous Mobility and Immobility in Migrant Healthcare along the US–Mexico Border 19
Heide Castañeda

Chapter 2 "It's Too Risky to Leave the House": Immigrant Policing and Health-Related Mobility 35
Nolan Kline

Chapter 3 (Im)mobile Populations and Health Rights: Accessing the Healthcare System in Slovenia 53
Uršula Lipovec Čebron and Sara Pistotnik

Part II. The Effect of Imagination on Mobility as a Resource in the Search for Care and Caring 73
Anne E. Pfister

Chapter 4 Fluid and Mobile Identities: Travel, Imaginaries, and Caregiving Practices among Families of Deaf Children in Mexico City 77
Anne E. Pfister and Cecilia Vindrola-Padros

Chapter 5 Egg Donor Social Mobility and Expansion of Czech Reproductive Medicine 99
Amy Speier

Chapter 6 Governing Mobility of Health Workers across Borders: From Local to Global Policy Tools 116
Evgeniya Plotnikova

Part III. Patient Navigation and Mobile Technologies of Care 139
Ginger A. Johnson

Chapter 7 HIV/AIDS and Voluntary Counseling and Testing (VCT) Services for Deaf Kenyans 143
Alina Engelman

Chapter 8 Service-Learning Research Projects to Enhance the Information Accompanying Commonly Dispensed Medicines on the Phelophepa Healthcare Trains 164
Sunitha C. Srinivas and Sharli A. Paphitis

Chapter 9 Community-Led Peer Advocacy for Transgender Healthcare Access in the Southeastern United States: The Trans Buddy Program 185
E. Kale Edmiston

Chapter 10 Leading mHealth in Myanmar's Smartphone Revolution 202
Perrie Briskin and Sara Lucía Gallo

Postscript 224
Cecilia Vindrola-Padros, Ginger A. Johnson, and Anne E. Pfister

Index 229

Figures and Tables

Figure 4.1 Image of the Mexico City Metro taken by Leo, an IPPLIAP student, during his commute to school. Photo courtesy of Leo. 79

Figure 6.1 Governance framework for the regulation of cross-border health worker mobility. 124

Figure 6.2 NMC initial registrations of migrant nurses (overseas and EEA), 1998–99 to 2013–14. 127

Figure 7.1 Tailor-made, accessible HIV/AIDS education message in Kenyan Sign Language (KSL) at a Deaf VCT site: "Together We Will Eradicate AIDS." 11 June 2006. 148

Figure 7.2 Tailor-made accessible HIV/AIDS education message in Kenyan Sign Language (KSL) at a Deaf VCT site, featuring an image of a grandmother holding a baby: "I'm glad my grandchild is HIV/AIDS free. My son and his wife went for HIV counseling and testing before having this baby." 11 June 2006. 150

Figure 7.3 Kichakamkwaju Primary School students seated outside waiting for a participatory theater performance to begin in which students acted out the role of a Deaf HIV+ person, a VCT counselor, and a hearing family member. 19 July 2006. 152

Figure 8.1 Ibuprofen pictographic MIL developed by third-year pharmacy students. 175

Figure 8.2 Chlorpheniramine pictographic MIL developed by third-year pharmacy students. 175

Figure 8.3 Disprin pictographic MIL developed by third-year pharmacy students. 176

Figure 9.1	Transphobic healthcare systems limit mobility and access.	192
Figure 10.1	Screenshots of maymay 1.0, released in September 2014.	209
Figure 10.2	Screenshots of maymay 2.0, released January 2016. This version added quizzes and articles to engage users.	211
Figure 10.3	Screenshots of maymay update, released in 2017. App now includes a Facebook-style newsfeed for users to scroll through.	212
Table 6.1	Changes to the foreign nurse registration process, immigration rules, and employment requirements since 2005	128

Introduction

Healthcare in Motion

Cecilia Vindrola-Padros, Ginger A. Johnson, and Anne E. Pfister

(Im)mobilities permeate every aspect of our daily life, including our opportunities, lifestyle choices, well-being, and access to healthcare. The scale of movement associated with obtaining health services is increasing, with an estimated five million people traveling to obtain medical care in another country (Horsfall and Lunt 2016). Healthcare professionals are also increasingly mobile, and it is estimated that low- and middle-income countries (LMICs) contribute between 40 and 75 percent of medical graduates to high-income countries (HICs), a phenomenon leading to "brain drain" in areas of the world with the highest levels of disease burden (Bradby 2014; Humphries et al. 2015; Mackey and Liang 2012; Mpofu, Sen Gupta, and Hays 2016). Healthcare practice is also becoming mobile with the incorporation of new technologies that adjust to patients' mobility trends through the use of devices (e.g., mHealth, or "mobile health"), in some cases, allowing the delivery of services without being in the same location (e.g., virtual healthcare services) (Fiordelli, Diviani, and Schulz 2013). In 2013 alone, approximately one thousand mHealth projects were implemented across the globe, and 65 percent of those were taking place in developing countries (Al Dahdah, Du Loû, and Méadel 2015; GSMA 2013).

The current state of movement of patients, healthcare professionals, and medical services opens opportunities to new forms of healthcare or higher quality of services for some populations, but limits access to care for others (Chen and Flood 2013; Whittaker, Manderson, and Cartwright 2010). As some populations become more mobile, others might face restrictions in movement as borders solidify, political tensions between "citizens" and "migrants" erupt, and policies dictating "deservingness" to public services are enforced (Messina 2011; Winton 2015). Technologies designed to empower healthcare users and disseminate health information to a wider range of stakeholders might remain available to the few groups able to access them (Al Dahdah et al. 2015). These differences in capacities for movement are the product of larger social, political, economic, and cultural factors that contribute to inequalities in the distribution of health services, and differences in the quality of available healthcare (Lee, Kearns, and Friesen 2010).

The turn toward a focus on mobilities in the social sciences has demonstrated the centrality of mobilities in our everyday lives (Salazar 2016) and draws our attention to the multiple ways in which being mobile (or immobile) is the product of individually negotiated social, cultural, economic, and political processes (Büscher and Urry 2009; Urry 2002; Urry 2007). As D'Andrea, Ciolfi, and Gray (2011: 150) have argued, "mobilities deserve to be examined in their own singularity, centrality and contingent determination, as they may destabilize and recode social and natural formations in ways that cannot be properly understood through the lenses of classical (sedentary) social theory." Movement and stasis can therefore be used as a window into social constructions of gender, class, ability, ethnicity, the cultural meaning of place, and identity formation, as well as experiences of delivering and obtaining health services and other forms of care.

Not all movement is the same and not all movement is voluntary (Hannam, Sheller, and Urry 2006). The analysis of the restriction or promotion of movement by healthcare policies and practices and the new modalities of healthcare that are shaped by emerging mobility forms allows us to explore the social and cultural construction of both mobility and healthcare. The movement required for obtaining health services can therefore take on different meanings than movement used for other purposes, as these journeys might be perceived and experienced as "healing," "restorative," and even "life-sparing." The geographies of medical spaces can simultaneously welcome or deter patients (Neuwelt, Kearns, and Browne 2015) and ultimately shape individual experiences of receiving health services and other forms of care in material (e.g., physical access) as well as emotional ways (Ergler et al. 2011). Clinical spaces can also function in both effective and affective ways, becoming places of treatment (focused on clinical outcomes), as well as therapeutic landscapes (focused on offering comfort and tranquility that may facilitate healing and well-being) (Lee et al. 2010). In the process of entering and navigating these medical spaces, people acquire additional roles (patient, healthcare professional, carer, etc.), and their movement might be organized in relation to predetermined clinical pathways that can be flexible and negotiated to some extent, but nonetheless set the roadmap for patient flows.

In the same way that healthcare policies and institutions shape mobility forms, new trends in (im)mobility redefine healthcare systems and what it means to be a patient, a carer, or a healthcare professional. As Kangas (2010: 357) has argued, "care takes on new meanings and obligations in today's interconnected world when consciences cannot settle for what is available locally." Treatment and health service labor mirror global capital flows as new and less expensive forms of travel can expand an ill person's sense of viable treatment options, leading them and their family to travel great distances to access what they consider to be the best type of care (Kangas 2007, 2010; Vindrola-Padros and Brage 2017). Potential employment opportunities located elsewhere in the world can foster the migration of healthcare professionals seeking better jobs and chances for career development. In the era of increasingly mobile healthcare, new actors—such as mobile network operators, technology developers, data management companies, and medical-tourism marketing experts—come into play and influence how health services are designed and delivered. Physical proximity is replaced by virtual platforms, potentially redefining the ways in which medicine is conceived and practiced (Ahlin 2013; Al Dahdah et al. 2015) and expanding our traditional notions of the need for co-presence (Urry 2002) in clinical encounters to include more remote ways of knowing and healing.

A significant amount of research has examined the migration of patients, health workers, and mobile health technologies, but further work needs to be carried out to understand processes of healthcare delivery within the context of (im)mobilities. *Healthcare in Motion* seeks to explore the dynamic interrelationship between mobility and healthcare by analyzing how gradients of movement and stasis interact to engender multiple forms of travel as people seek or deliver health services. The book is guided by the following questions: (1) How does the need to obtain and deliver health services engender particular (im)mobility forms? (2) How is mobility experienced and imagined when it is required for healthcare access or delivery?

The focus on ground-level, subjective experiences of mobility and healthcare allows the authors in this volume to study and understand mobility as a social practice imbued with cultural meaning, thus gaining insight into the social, cultural, political, and economic processes that make mobility possible as well as those that restrict movement. Most of the authors apply frameworks and perspectives stemming from the social sciences, but several are also practitioners who design or deliver health services on the ground and can shed light on the day-to-day practices of moving health services closer to the people who need them. Mobility and healthcare are represented as complex cultural and political processes, which are not only influenced by global policies and structures, but also shaped daily by individuals and their local communities.

Structure of the Book

The book is divided into three main sections: (1) Healthcare and differential mobility empowerments; (2) Mobility as a resource in the search for care and caring; and (3) Patient navigation and mobile technologies of care. The three sections cover important areas of health and healthcare understood in relation to different types of mobility forms. Each section contains a short preface that serves as an introduction to the main concepts and approaches discussed in the chapters in the section. The chapters—written by authors from various disciplines, including anthropology, social policy, philosophy, nursing, pharmacy, public health, and neuroscience—draw from experiences and case studies taking place in geographical and cultural contexts such as the United States, Mexico, Kenya, South Africa, Myanmar, Slovenia, and the Czech Republic.

Healthcare and Differential Mobility Empowerments

Not everyone who wants to use mobility as a resource is able to do so (Morley 2002; Skeggs 2004). As Tesfahuney (1998: 501) has argued, "differential mobility empowerments reflect structures and hierarchies of power and position by race, gender, age and class, ranging from the local and the global." This section engages explicitly with the ways in which public policies create and reproduce these "differential mobility empowerments," where some groups are represented as "deserving" of free movement and access to public services, while others are contained and not considered eligible for services as essential as healthcare.

The chapters by Nolan Kline and Heide Castañeda address this topic in the United States. Kline explores the relationship between immigration policies, mobility, and healthcare, demonstrating the effects of immigrant policing on health-seeking behaviors and access to medical services. In his ethnographic research in Atlanta, Georgia, Kline found that undocumented immigrants avoid visiting medical facilities due to the fear of deportation. The risk of deportation is perceived not only in clinics, but also while driving to obtain medical services or participate in daily activities, such as commuting to work. Migrants thus perceive and experience constant threats to their lifestyle and well-being and adapt their mobility accordingly. While exploring these processes through the lens of automobility, Kline argues that current US immigration policies underlie health inequalities by creating structural vulnerabilities and inequalities in movement that prevent undocumented migrants from maintaining their health and seeking medical attention.

Castañeda's chapter deals with undocumented migrants' experiences of accessing health services in the Texas/Mexico borderlands, arguing that they are "stuck in motion." Bordering processes in the United States constrain the movement of undocumented migrants to the extent that they feel in a constant state of "stuckness." This idea alludes to both fixity and motion, and is an attempt to consider the coexistence of mobility and immobility without succumbing to the restrictions of the movement/stasis dichotomy (Khan 2016). Mobilities and moorings intertwine to produce instances of stillness, fixity, and restraint (Hannam et al. 2006), but being stuck does not mean being immobile. The migrants Castañeda worked with shared the diverse strategies they use to negotiate borders, both lived and imagined, and restrictions in movement to obtain medical services, restore their health, and, in some cases, save the lives of their children. According to Castañeda, if we shift our conceptualization of borders from a fence or a wall to the stillness of people, we might be able to rethink borders as dynamic and inhabited places, places that change, have meaning, and matter.

Uršula Lipovec Čebron and Sara Pistotnik also explore the relationship between public policies and healthcare access by discussing the case of "the erased" in Slovenia. The erased were citizens of former Yugoslav republics who either did not apply for residency after the Slovenian independence or had their applications rejected. Despite former residence in the country, they were erased from national registries and lost access to public services, including most healthcare services, equating their status with that of undocumented migrants. They became classified as an "undeserving population" and entered a state of liminality, where they remained fixated in the same physical space but without being able to enforce their social and political rights. As Khan (2016: 98) has argued, "liminality is inflected in the broader political-economic condition of not moving, and never arriving," and thus, as a concept, allows us to glimpse the experience of being and feeling immobile. These new health policies first excluded "the erased" and other migrants, but different forms of restricted access to health services are experienced contemporarily by a rising number of residents, especially after the 2008 economic crisis.

Mobility as a Resource in the Search for Care and Caring

Experts studying mobility among human populations expose a provocative juxtaposition regarding who travels and why. Scholars agree that mobility is not a new phenomenon among humans (Urry 2002; Salazar and Smart 2011), that mobility is "basic to human social life" (Glick Schiller and Salazar 2013: 184), and that, for many, being on the move has become a way of life (Urry 2000; Urry 2002). Yet scholars increasingly recognize the inequity of *motility,* or the ability or potential to move (Kaufmann, Bergman, and Joyce 2004; Leivestad 2016). Research in many disciplines reveals stark and subtle ways that motility, as a potential resource employed to solve basic human problems, is not equally accessible to all members of societies, nor equitably distributed globally (Salazar and Smart 2011). Capacities for movement are framed by global policies and the local context, but also negotiated by individuals in their daily practices.

The endeavor of section two is the exploration of these individual experiences of movement and the corresponding narratives revealing why people seek movement as a resource. The authors in this section explore physical acts of movement as well as what Lean, Staiff, and Waterton (2014) have referred to as "imaginaries" of travel—or the effect of imagination on potential and performed travel experiences. Attention to these imaginaries of travel reveals the creativity that people employ as they seek mobility as a resource to solve problems related to health and healthcare.

Anne E. Pfister and Cecilia Vindrola-Padros describe the movement of families of deaf children in and around Mexico City. The journey upon which these families embarked following deaf diagnoses compelled them to find ways of understanding their children's deafness, and as they did, their identities were refashioned in ways they could not have imagined. These families, in their quest for information and assistance, engaged in what Urry (2002) refers to as *corporeal* travel, or movement that explicitly involves bodies in motion. The physical movement of these families as they sought care is the most obvious component of their mobility. However, their simultaneous movement through stages of identity formation—how they imagined and reimagined themselves as parents of deaf children—accompanied and, in some cases, transcended physical movement and was ultimately the most transformational component of their travel.

Amy Speier explores the experiences of women who participate in the reproductive travel industry in the Czech Republic. This study is part of a growing body of literature documenting the expansion of the medical-tourism industry and scholarly contemplation of its potential implications (Chen and Flood 2013; Kangas 2010; Whittaker and Speier 2010). Through careful contextualization and the honesty of her ethnographic participants, Speier reveals how regional, social, economic, and imagined movements impact young, childless Czech women and women on maternity leave. Her exposition links the accessibility of new and flexible types of financial gain—via egg donation—with the perception among this population of social and cultural mobility through their reproductive choices. Again, physical movement (of intended parents as tourists, of egg donors) becomes the backdrop as we learn about the complex inner negotiations of the egg donors and consider the consequences of the services they offer.

Evgeniya Plotnikova explores the global mobility of health workers by drawing our attention to the interaction of economic factors, policy and regulation, and individual practices impacting their mobility. She offers insight into the challenges of regulating health worker mobility, offering examples of the "complex and multilevel character of contemporary migration," composed of multisited migration routes with a final desired (and ultimately imagined) destination to which individuals cling throughout these extended journeys. Plotnikova asks: What policies can adequately manage health worker migration, secure access to health services in source countries, and protect migrant health workers from the risk of exploitation and from racial and gender discrimination in receiving countries? Policy tools attempting to regulate cross-border health workers are the focus of this chapter, yet we are drawn into the examples Plotnikova provides and are reminded that global policies are not always attuned to the individual creativity and imaginaries of health workers that ultimately affect their mobility.

Patient Navigation and Mobile Technologies of Care

In global context, health disparities between rural and urban populations are stark and this gap continues to widen, with rapid social and economic transformations creating adverse effects in health that "disproportionately affect the poorest and most disadvantaged" (UNICEF 2015: 3). However, utilization of healthcare services is not only about "getting there," but also about how patient-provider interactions are guided (or not) once "there." As stated above, mobilities literature focuses not only on the barriers that may (im)mobilize patients and healthcare providers, but also on the quality of available healthcare services and how that care affects patient and user experiences. These barriers might deter patients from obtaining treatment or effectively adhering to medical advice (Ensor and Cooper 2004).

In low- and middle-income countries, these barriers are more likely to affect the poor, while in wealthier nations they are most pronounced among socially vulnerable and marginalized groups (Ensor and Cooper 2004). Mobile healthcare solutions, including mHealth initiatives, have the potential to address many of the challenges faced by under-resourced health systems, particularly with regard to linking rural and hard-to-reach populations with health facilitators (e.g., community health workers) and urban health professionals (Marshall, Lewis, and Whittaker 2013; Mishra and Singh 2008).

The authors in this section seek to describe and critically examine the implementation of health interventions aimed at addressing barriers to healthcare access. The chapters in this section cover three continents and a range of health issues, from HIV/AIDS among the deaf and hard-of-hearing in Kenya to family planning and reproductive, maternal and child health services in Myanmar. Yet, the common thread throughout each of the unique ethnographic case studies presented here are descriptions of health interventions that seek to (1) utilize new or existing infrastructures to bring patients and healthcare providers together and (2) guide the appropriate translation of health information from provider to patient.

The chapter by Alina Engelman discusses the barriers to HIV/AIDS education and services in receiving care that are faced by deaf and hard-of-hearing Kenyans who are HIV-positive or living with AIDS—a population often immobilized by the inability to effectively communicate with family, friends, peers, and program staff. LVCT Health is an indigenous nonprofit, nongovernmental organization in Kenya serving at-risk populations including men who have sex with men, prisoners and sex workers, and the deaf. Its programming includes community-based mobile voluntary counseling and testing (VCT) outreach services and participatory theater in rural areas. After mobilizing VCT units to reach populations in need, three critical components of the deaf program trained members of the deaf community to provide peer-based HIV/AIDS education and services, putting deaf Kenyans in key leadership roles in VCT sites throughout Kenya, and teaching hearing HIV and sexual health service providers basic Kenyan Sign Language to enable their effective communication with patients. Engelman's chapter describes a program evaluation and needs assessment of LVCT Health to provide recommendations for program improvement and, ultimately, to demonstrate "the empowering nature of community-driven healthcare delivery." The author concludes by exploring the ways in which mHealth can enhance the mission of LVCT Health.

Sunitha C. Srinivas and Sharli A. Paphitis describe the physical and informational barriers to basic healthcare services that affect patients in impoverished areas of rural South Africa. Two South African trains currently operate as mobile clinics to increase patient access to basic healthcare in underserved rural areas. To increase the rational use of medicines among the illiterate populations served by the mobile clinic, South African education institutions such as Rhodes University provide service-learning opportunities for pharmacy students to design medicine information leaflets that embody cultural appropriateness, readability, and understanding for a low-literate population. Service-learning opportunities serve to introduce students to the challenges healthcare workers face in delivering healthcare and the challenges patients face in attempting to comply with medical advice. Ultimately, this opportunity serves to train a future generation of healthcare professionals "to be more aware of and responsive to a broader range of societal health care needs."

The chapter by E. Kale Edmiston explores the health and healthcare inequalities experienced by transgender persons living in the US South. These inequalities include discriminatory (and potentially dangerous) politically partisan legislation that restricts movement in public spaces, higher rates of violence (including murder), higher rates of HIV/AIDS, and mental health concerns. In response, the Trans Buddy Program is a unique program founded in Nashville, Tennessee, to improve mobility of and healthcare access by transgender persons by providing volunteer peer advocates. These "buddies" offer phone support, including health referrals and resources, and may provide in-person support by, for example, attending healthcare appointments with patients. Because many transgender persons in the South have limited access to local care and may have limited mobility, the Trans Buddy Program helps to circumvent some of their needs for physical mobility by providing support services over the phone (a deliberately low-tech solution) and, when requested, by supporting transgender patients in navigating rigid healthcare systems that often do not take into consideration the unique health needs of transgender identities and bodies.

Perrie Briskin and Sara Lucía Gallo discuss new technological channels for virtually reaching out to women of reproductive age in Myanmar—a country with low contraceptive use and high maternal mortality—with key messages on family planning and reproductive, maternal, and child health. Within this context, Population Services International launched the first-ever maternal health mobile smartphone app in Myanmar (called "maymay") in recognition of the country's rapidly changing digital landscape. The maymay app (downloaded more than sixty thousand times as of May 2016) allows women to privately access key family planning and reproductive health messaging, in addition to an extensive medical provider network. The multiple rounds of testing, modifying, and evaluating the app for user acceptability that maymay has undergone since its early development and initial launch in 2014 serve as an important reminder that the delivery of health information—whether virtually or in person—must be responsive to the needs of its intended audience. As stated by the authors, digital health initiatives must seek to "ensure that messages remain relevant and that target populations remain tuned in."

Concluding Remarks

Health, healthcare, and the practice of caring are currently being reconfigured by increased flows of patients, healthcare workers, and medical technologies. In response to this increased mobility, scholarly attention turns toward related stigmas, inequities, political ideologies, and policies that delineate populations as "deserving" and "non-deserving" of health-related services. The interconnection between (im)mobilities and healthcare is therefore an area ripe for analysis and critical exploration. The chapters within this book highlight the need to focus on the particularities of the experiences of movement and stasis when attempting to explore the broader interconnection between (im)mobilities and healthcare. As people move, their bodies (racialized, gendered, aged, classed, impaired, sexualized, or (un)healthy) shape how, when, where, and if they move (Büscher and Urry 2009). This book is a pioneering attempt that acknowledges these particularities while exploring the experience of movement in the context of healthcare access and delivery. Collectively, these chapters contribute to mobility studies, as an emerging field of inquiry, and prompt further exploration of healthcare (im)mobilities.

Cecilia Vindrola-Padros, PhD, is a research associate in the Department of Applied Health Research, University College London, UK. A medical anthropologist, she has researched the experiences of children and families who relocate to access medical treatment. Recent publications on mobility include the book chapters "Children Seeking Health Care: International Perspectives on Children's Use of Mobility to Obtain Health Services" (with Ginger Johnson), in *Movement, Mobilities, and Journeys: Geographies of Children and Young People* (Springer, 2017), and "Child Medical Travel in Argentina: Narratives of Family Separation and Moving Away from Home" (with Eugenia Brage), in *Children's Health and Wellbeing in Urban Environments* (Routledge, 2017).

Ginger A. Johnson, PhD, is a visiting assistant professor at Southern Methodist University. She holds a PhD in medical anthropology and a master's degree in global public health from the University of South Florida and a master's degree in international law from the United Nations Interregional Crime and Justice Research Institute. Recently, she was embedded in West Africa conducting Ebola-related research with the International Federation of the Red Cross. A selection of her current research projects includes addressing adolescent nutritional needs in Cambodia, for the World Food Programme, and ensuring social accountability for maternal and child health in Malawi, for UNICEF.

Anne E. Pfister, PhD, is assistant professor of anthropology at the University of North Florida. Her research investigates how deaf youth and their families experience deafness in Mexico City, by integrating sociocultural linguistic theory with biocultural medical anthropology analyses. Her current project utilizes visual methods, including "photovoice," to actively engage participants as co-researchers. She has been involved with the Mexican deaf community for over ten years. Her research interests include disabilities studies, language socialization, and medicalization; her work has been published in *Ethos*, *Visual Anthropology Review*, *Behavioral and Brain Sciences*, *Collaborative Anthropologies*, and *Annals of Anthropological Practice*.

REFERENCES

Ahlin, T. 2013. "Is There an App for That? Anthropology Takes the Pulse of E-health." *Second Opinion—Society for Medical Anthropology* 1(4): 7–8.

Al Dahdah, M., A. Du Loû, and C. Méadel. 2015. "Mobile Health and Maternal Care: A Winning Combination for Healthcare in the Developing World?" *Health Policy and Technology* 4(3): 225–231.

Bradby, H. 2014. "International Medical Migration: A Critical Conceptual Review of the Global Movement of Doctors and Nurses." *Health* 18(6): 580–596.

Büscher, M., and J. Urry. 2009. "Mobile Methods and the Empirical." *European Journal of Social Theory* 12(1): 99–116.

Chen, Y., and C. Flood. 2013. "Medical Tourism's Impact on Health Care Equity and Access in Low- and Middle-Income Countries: Making the Case for Regulation." *Journal of Law, Medicine and Ethics* 41(1): 286–300.

D'Andrea, A., L. Ciolfi, and B. Gray. 2011. "Methodological Challenges and Innovations in Mobilities Research." *Mobilities* 6(2): 149–160.

Ensor, T., and S. Cooper. 2004. "Overcoming Barriers to Health Service Access: Influencing the Demand Side." *Health Policy and Planning* 19(2): 69–79.

Ergler, C., P. Sakdapolrak, H. Bohle, and R. Kearns. 2011. "Entitlements to Health Care: Why Is There a Preference for Private Facilities among Poorer Residents of Chennai, India?" *Social Science & Medicine* 72(3): 327–337.

Fiordelli, M., N. Diviani, and P. Schulz. 2013. "Mapping mHealth Research: A Decade of Evolution." *Journal of Medical Internet Research* 15(5): e95.

Glick Schiller, N., and N. B. Salazar. 2013. "Regimes of Mobility across the Globe." *Journal of Ethnic and Migration Studies* 39(2): 183–200.

GSMA. 2013. The GSMA mHealth Tracker. Retrieved 29 March 2018 from https://www.gsma.com/mobilefordevelopment/m4d-tracker/mhealth-deployment-tracker.

Hannam, K., M. Sheller, and J. Urry. 2006. "Editorial: Mobilites, Immobilities and Moorings." *Mobilities* 1(1): 1–22.

Horsfall, D., and N. Lunt (2016). "Medical Tourism by Numbers." In *Handbook on Medical Tourism and Patient Mobility,* ed. N. Lunt, D. Horsfall, and J. Hanefled, 25–36. Cheltenham, UK: Edward Elgar.

Humphries, N., S. McAleese, A. Matthews, and R. Brugha. 2015. "'Emigration is a matter of self-preservation. The working conditions . . . are killing us slowly': Qualitative Insights into Health Professional Emigration from Ireland." *Human Resources for Health* 13: 35.

Kangas, B. 2007. "Hope from Abroad in the International Medical Travel of Yemeni Patients." *Anthropology and Medicine* 14(3): 293–305.

Kangas, B. 2010. "Traveling for Medical Care in a Global World." *Medical Anthropology* 29(4): 344–362.

Kaufmann, V., M. Bergman, and D. Joyce. 2004. "Motility: Mobility as Capital." *International Journal of Urban and Regional Research* 28(4): 745–756.

Khan, N. 2016. "Immobility." In *Keywords of Mobility: Critical Engagements,* ed. N. Salazar and K. Jayaram, 93–112. Oxford, UK: Berghahn Books.

Lean, G., R. Staiff, and E. Waterton. 2014. *Travel and Imagination.* Farnham, UK: Ashgate Publishing.

Lee, J. Y., R. A. Kearns, and W. Friesen. 2010. "Seeking Affective Health Care: Korean Immigrants' Use of Homeland Medical Services." *Health & Place* 16(1): 108–115.

Leivestad, H. 2016. "Motility." In *Keywords of Mobility: Critical Engagements,* ed. N. Salazar and K. Jayaram, 133–151. Oxford, UK: Berghahn Books.

Mackey, T., and B. Liang. 2012. "Rebalancing Brain Drain: Exploring Resource Reallocation to Address Health Worker Migration and Promote Global Health." *Health Policy* 107(1): 66–73.

Marshall, C., D. Lewis, and M. Whittaker. (2013). "mHealth Technologies in Developing Countries: A Feasibility Assessment and a Proposed Framework." Health Information Systems Knowledge Hub, Working Paper Series, No. 25. Herston, Australia: School of Population Health, University of Queensland.

Messina, A. M. 2011. "Asylum, Residency and Citizenship Policies and Models of Migrant Incorporation." In *Migration and Health in the European Union,* ed. B. Rechel, P. Mladovsky, W. Devillé, B. Rijks, R. Petrova-Benedict, and M. McKee, 37–51. Berkshire, England: McGraw Hill/Open University Press.

Mishra, S., and I. P. Singh. (2008). "mHealth: A Developing Country Perspective." Global Partnerships, Local Solutions Conference, Bellagio, 13 July–8 August 2008. Bellagio, Italy: Making the eHealth Connection.

Morley, D. 2002. *Home Territories: Media, Mobility and Identity.* London: Routledge.

Mpofu C., T. Sen Gupta, and R. Hays. 2016. "The Ethics of Medical Practitioner Migration from Low-Resourced Countries to the Developed World: A Call for Action by Health Systems and Individual Doctors." *Journal of Bioethical Inquiry* 13(3): 395–406.

Neuwelt, P., R. A. Kearns, and A. Browne. 2015. "The Place of Receptionists in Access to Primary Care: Challenges in the Space between Community and Consultation." *Social Science & Medicine* 133: 287–295.

Pathy, V. 2012. Harmonizing Supply and Demand for Health Care Services: An Exploration of Demand-Based Strategies to Encourage the Active Engagement of Consumers. Report. Denver, CO: Center for Improving Value in Health Care.

Salazar, N. 2016. "Keywords of Mobility: What's in a Name?" In *Keywords of Mobility: Critical Engagements,* ed. N. Salazar and K. Jayaram, 1–12. Oxford, UK: Berghahn Books.

Salazar, N. B., and A. Smart. 2011. "Anthropological Takes on (Im)mobility." *Identities: Global Studies in Culture and Power* 18(6): i–ix.

Shea, B., N. Andersson, and D. Henry. 2009. "Increasing the Demand for Childhood Vaccination in Developing Countries: A Systematic Review." *BMC International Health and Human Rights* 9(Suppl. 1): S5. doi:10.1186/1472-698X-9-S1-S5.

Skeggs, B. 2004. *Class, Self, Culture.* London: Routledge.

Stolley, K. S., and S. Watson. 2012. *Medical Tourism: A Reference Handbook.* Santa Barbara, CA: ABC-CLIO.

Tesfahuney, M. 1998. "Mobility, Racism and Geopolitics." *Political Geography* 17(5): 499–515.
UNICEF (United Nations Children's Fund). 2015. *For Every Child, a Fair Chance: The Promise of Equity.* New York: UNICEF. Retrieved 28 October 2016 from http://www.unicef.org/publications/files/For_every_child_a_fair_chance.pdf.
Urry, J. 2000. *Sociology beyond Societies.* London: Routledge.
———. 2002. "Mobility and Proximity." *Sociology* 36(2): 255–274.
———. 2007. *Mobilities.* Cambridge, UK: Polity Press.
Vindrola-Padros, C., and E. Brage. 2017. "Child Medical Travel in Argentina: Narratives of Family Separation and Moving Away from Home." In *Children's Health and Well-being in Urban Environments,* ed. C. R. Ergler and R. A. Kearnes. New York: Routledge.
Whittaker, A., and A. Speier. 2010. "'Cycling Overseas': Care, Commodification, and Stratification in Cross-Border Reproductive Travel." *Medical Anthropology* 29(4): 363–83.
Whittaker, A., L. Manderson, and E. Cartwright. 2010. "Patients without Borders: Understanding Medical Travel." *Medical Anthropology* 29(4): 336–343.
Winton, A. 2015. "Violence, Borders, and Boundaries: Reframing Young People's Mobility." In *Movement, Mobilities, and Journeys: Geographies of Children and Young People,* ed. C.N. Laoire, A. White, and T. Skelton, 1–19. Singapore: Springer.

PART I

Healthcare and Differential Mobility Empowerments

Cecilia Vindrola-Padros

> The unwelcome migrant not only faces the prospect of an increasingly treacherous border crossing, but also having to negotiate a highly complex, contradictory barrage of institutions, authorities and criminals on the other side, wishing to variously deport, assist or exploit them.
>
> —Ailsa Winton, "Violence, Borders, and Boundaries"

The three chapters in this section explore the interconnections between migration, immobility, and healthcare. The authors use ethnographic examples from the United States and Slovenia to illustrate the tangible effects of exclusionary migration policies on the health and well-being of "undocumented" migrants and "erased" populations. These policies operate on the ground, trickle into all aspects of daily life, and mark their migrant bodies as unwanted and, therefore, undeserving of medical services (Parrini et al. 2007: 62). Their demarcation as "different from others" is the product of the politics of embodiment that continuously (re)constructs their bodies and permeates experiences of movement and stasis (Jackson 2015: 2; Parrini et al. 2007).

The lives of the migrants described by Castañeda, Kline, and Lipovec and Pistotnik traverse through multiple, and often overlapping, states of movement and immobility, highlighting the structures created locally to constrain their movement as well as the ways in which migrants chisel through those structures to obtain care. Migrants attempting to obtain medical attention go through temporary states of immobility or "stuckness" (a term proposed in Castañeda's chapter) while grappling with the liminality of their status and the process of waiting for care (see also Khan 2016). The conceptual space created by waiting is a useful analytical tool for examining power relations and inequalities in care as those who wait are often in more vulnerable positions (Conlon 2011: 355).

The richness of the migrant experience as described by the authors in this section was generated through the use of mobile ethnographic methods, allowing researchers to "ride along," "walk with," and immerse themselves in the daily lives of undocumented migrants and the healthcare professionals they encounter. These ethnographic perspectives make important contributions to the study of (im)mobilities and healthcare as they allow the researcher to examine movement across multiple locales and scales, in time, in practice, and in the imagination (Dalakoglou and Harvey 2012). Mobility is theorized as a complex social process, entailing different modalities and layers of movement (Chalfin 2016), and access to healthcare is critically examined to uncover the relations of power and structural inequalities that guarantee high-quality services for some and deny them to others (Willen, Mulligan, and Castañeda 2011).

Discussion Questions

In reading through the chapters in this section, it may be useful to keep the following questions in mind:

1. How do migration policies frame undocumented migrants' interaction with the healthcare system?
2. How do migrants negotiate and bypass movement restrictions?
3. What are the different forms of immobility experienced by undocumented migrants seeking healthcare services?

REFERENCES

Chalfin, B. 2016. "Multiple Mobilities and the Ethnographic Engagement of Keywords." In *Keywords of Mobility: Critical Engagements*, ed. N. Salazar and K. Jayaram, 171–77. Oxford, UK: Berghahn Books.

Conlon, D. 2011. "Waiting: Feminist Perspectives on the Spacings/Timings of Migrant (Im)mobility." *Gender, Place and Culture* 18(3): 353–360.

Dalakoglou, D., and P. Harvey. 2012. "Roads and Anthropology: Ethnographic Perspectives on Space, Time and (Im)mobility." *Mobilities* 7(4): 459–465.

Jackson, L. 2015. "Experiencing Exclusion and Reacting to Stereotypes? Navigating Borders of the Migrant Body." *Area* 48(3): 292–299.

Khan, N. 2016. "Immobility." In *Keywords of Mobility: Critical Engagements,* ed. N. Salazar and K. Jayaram, 93–112. Oxford, UK: Berghahn Books.

Parrini, R., X. Castañeda, C. Magis, J. Ruiz, and G. Lemp. 2007. "Migrant Bodies: Corporality, Sexuality, and Power among Mexican Migrant Men." *Sexuality Research and Social Policy* 4(3): 62–73.

Willen, S., J. Mulligan, and H. Castañeda. 2011. "Take a Stand Commentary: How Can Medical Anthropologists Contribute to Contemporary Conversations on 'Illegal' Im/migration and Health?" *Medical Anthropology Quarterly* 25(3): 331–356.

Winton, A. 2015. "Violence, Borders, and Boundaries: Reframing Young People's Mobility." In *Movement, Mobilities, and Journeys, Geographies of Children and Young People,* ed. C. N. Laoire, A. White, and T. Skelton, 1–19. Singapore: Springer.

CHAPTER 1

"Stuck in Motion"

Simultaneous Mobility and Immobility in Migrant Healthcare along the US–Mexico Border

Heide Castañeda

> It's just immoral for us as a society to expect a mother to stay behind while her eight-year-old daughter has to travel four hundred miles away for treatment. To tell her, "No, you're not allowed to go." In what world is that all right?
> —Community health center physician, Hidalgo County, Texas

Both mobility and healthcare are complex cultural and sociopolitical processes, influenced by policies and structures but also shaped on the ground in local communities. The new mobilities paradigm has focused on the social meanings attached to movement and their relationship to frameworks of power, indicating that mobility is an unevenly distributed resource. Beyond the production of movement, and how particular modes of such are enabled, we must also be attentive to mobilities that are "forbidden, regulated, policed, and prevented" (Cresswell 2006: 735). In other words, mobilities also beget immobilities, and are accompanied by particular social exclusions (Hannam, Sheller, and Urry 2006).

Borders represent the ultimate regulation of mobility, creating uneven landscapes of movement. The convergence of critical migration and mobility studies has focused on the ways in which some mobilities are facilitated while others are restricted (Winton 2015) and how the two are bound together by an "embodied politics of difference" (Blunt 2007: 2). Migration studies have been useful in countering sedentist approaches prominent in the social sciences, which treat stability and place as normal, and have highlighted issues of dislocation, disjuncture, and zones of social exclusion in the study of mobility (Sheller and Urry 2006).

This chapter explores the contradictory processes by which mobility associated with healthcare access is both fostered and hindered in communities along the US-Mexico border. I argue that people living in this dynamic region—characterized by historical patterns of migration, rapid population growth, and cross-border economic activity—also experience extreme restrictions in mobility, making it difficult to access healthcare services in all directions and at multiple scales.

Following an overview of the US-Mexico borderlands, I turn to a discussion of mixed mobility patterns within families and households that result from the policy intersections of health and immigration. Next, I describe why travel to other parts of the state or to the United States—necessary for some types of specialty medical care—is inaccessible to some residents of the region. At the same time, while cross-border care is a unique opportunity and notable feature of the area, it has become more restricted in recent years with increased militarization of the US-Mexico border. Finally, in the section "Mobile Medicines and Mobile Providers," I describe practices put into motion that have emerged in response to lack of mobility to obtain regular healthcare: the informal importation of Mexican medicines, unregulated pharmaceutical markets, medication sharing, and the rise of unlicensed medical and dental providers. This chapter concludes that in the borderlands context—which includes not only everyday surveillance and extreme poverty, but also resilience and high levels of informality—people become "stuck in motion," experiencing simultaneous mobility and immobility in attempts to access healthcare. As such, this case contributes to the study of mobilities as complex assemblages and experiences of movement that represent more than mere physical motion (Salazar, Elliot, and Norum 2017) and the ways in which people, places, and things—including healthcare resources—are linked to one another.

Methods

This chapter is informed by a five-year longitudinal ethnographic study of the healthcare landscape of the US-Mexico borderlands, specifically, the Lower Rio Grande Valley of South Texas. The project focused on mixed-status families, which contain varied constellations of citizens, permanent legal residents, undocumented immigrants, and individuals in legal limbo through temporary protected status or deferred action programs. These families now constitute a primary feature of the contemporary migration experience in the United States and offer a lens through which to examine the intersection of health and immigration policy (Castañeda 2017; Castañeda and Melo 2014). Here, I present some of the major themes that emerged related to mobility and healthcare access, informed by 252 semistructured interviews with individuals from mixed-status families. The interviews lasted between one and two hours and were typically conducted in the homes of participants, frequently because of participants' lack of (auto)mobility due to limitations associated with legal status, including poverty and, for those who are undocumented, the inability to procure a driver's license. The data from mixed-status families was supplemented by interviews with sixty-two healthcare providers, caseworkers, organizational staff, educators, and public health officials. This was further triangulated by extensive on-the-ground participant observation in communities and local medical settings across the five years of the study.

As with many studies of migration, even in such geographically enclosed spaces, this topic required that the researchers themselves be "on the move" (Sheller and Urry 2006). However, in dealing with experiences in a healthcare system, this also necessitated a consideration of scale (Salazar et al. 2017) and included both vertical scaling of methods—understanding deeply historical connections between local neighborhoods, border regions, and international migratory flows through longitudinal examination—and horizontal scaling in the form of multiple field sites, ranging from private homes to institutions such as medical clinics.

Mobilities and the US–Mexico Borderlands

The US-Mexico border features prominently in the regulation of mobility and remains an analytically powerful construct for examining historical patterns of inclusion and exclusion and the enduring territorial authority of the state in limiting mobility (Heyman 2008, 2010), despite increased surveillance and regulation in spaces of the nation's interior (Stuesse and Coleman 2014). The 2,000-mile border region is home to over 11.5 million people, many of whom reside in sister cities on either side of the international boundary. For centuries, transnational ties have created interdependent communities and linked forms of everyday life. In addition to early settlement patterns, transnational linkages have been fostered through interconnected economies and recent immigration flows (O'Leary and Sanchez 2011).

This region encapsulates a number of contradictions in regards to ethnonational identity, political participation, economic activity, education, and healthcare practices (Fleuriet and Castañeda 2017). The Texas-Mexico border is unique because of the geophysical separation created by the Rio Grande River and the resulting twenty-six bridges connecting the two countries. Even though many people cross the border daily for work, for recreation, and to visit family, this form of mobility is only available to some segments of the population. Undocumented persons who entered without inspection or have overstayed a visa are relegated to a small strip of land along the border, because they are also entrapped by secondary border policing practices. They are unable not only to cross back into Mexico (since they do not have authorization to re-enter the United States, where they now live), but also to travel to other parts of the United States because of the presence of US Customs and Border Protection (CBP) checkpoints along all major roads and highways. As a result, many individuals describe being "trapped" in the area even after living there for decades, and their Mexican town of origin—perhaps only a ten-minute drive—may feel hundreds of miles away.

Despite being a node of major international commercial activity, with billions of dollars flowing through it each day, this is one of the most disadvantaged areas of the United States, ranking last in per capita income. Many families reside in one of 2,300 *colonias*—unincorporated neighborhoods often lacking paved roads, water, electricity, and sewage systems. This region is considered one of the most medically underserved areas in the United States, due to a high uninsured rate, gaps in public health services, high rates of chronic disease, and pathogenic environmental concerns such as groundwater contamination and crowding. While the Rio Grande Valley has one of the highest uninsured rates in the nation, a large portion of the population remained ineligible for insurance or subsidies through the 2010 health care reform, because they either are not legal residents or earn less than 100 percent of the federal poverty level. These working poor were excluded by Texas's decision to not expand adult Medicaid, which would have insured an additional 1.5 million low-income adults. As a result, large numbers of uninsured individuals still persist in the region, and the severely underfunded local level is charged with trying to fill the gaps in healthcare services (Castañeda 2017a, Castañeda 2017b).

The centrality of migration for local communities in the US-Mexico borderlands cannot be overstated. In this region, about one-third of the population is foreign born, and 57 percent of children (most of whom are US citizens) live with at least one immigrant parent (Richardson and Pisani 2012). An estimated 89 percent of the population here is of Mexican descent, and Spanish is the preferred language for 90 percent of residents in the region (Mier et al. 2004). The range of health challenges associated with immigration is wide and often the result of the pathogenic role of social inequality (Castañeda et al. 2015; Willen, Mulligan, and Castañeda 2011). Immigration status affects health through mechanisms including fear, stress, differential access to resources, experiences of prejudice and violence, family separation, and differential access to safe work and housing (Castañeda et al. 2015). At the same time, eligibility for healthcare services is determined by legal status. The technicalities and practices of immigration and healthcare are intimately linked through processes of inspection and categorization.

Access to Care and Mixed Mobility Prospects within Families

Currently, there are an estimated 2.3 million mixed-status families in the United States (Passel 2011). These are families comprised of a mix of undocumented immigrants, citizens, permanent legal residents, and those with uncertain legal status (such as recipients of temporary protected status or deferred action). The majority of children in such families—an estimated 4.5 million—are US citizens by birth, representing three-quarters of all children of undocumented immigrants. These families are complex in regards to migrant status, legal documentation, and national identity and require a move beyond simple binaries of "authorized" and "unauthorized" to capture various dimensions of legal-status gray zones and ambiguity (Gonzales 2011; Suárez-Orozco et al. 2011).

Notably, the construction of "illegality" for parents and siblings influences opportunities for those who are US citizens, impacting their healthcare resources and social mobility (Castañeda and Melo 2014; Mangual Figueroa 2012; Menjívar and Abrego 2009; O'Leary and Sanchez 2011). Research shows that US citizen children with immigrant parents access programs such as Medicaid and the Children's Health Insurance Program (CHIP) at a lower rate than those with citizen parents (Hagan et al. 2003; Huang, Yu, and Ledsky 2006; Pereira et al. 2012). In addition, parents' fear of interacting with authorities because of the threat of deportation may lead them to limit or delay services for their children, even when they are entitled (Abrego and Menjívar 2011; Capps et al. 2004). In some cases, parents will withdraw their children from programs altogether (Xu and Brabeck 2012). Finally, if parents are able to apply for permanent residency status in the future, they will be assessed as to whether or not they represent a "public charge," that is, if they have been or will be dependent on the government. This has led to some families avoiding health services for eligible children, because they fear that it will affect future chances at regularization (Castañeda and Melo 2014; Mendoza 2009; Park 2011). When immigration and healthcare access policies are combined, an environment is created "in which immigrants are often ineligible, discouraged or frightened from obtaining public health insurance coverage and health care services" (Hagan et al. 2003: 459).

Unauthorized children and parents, on the other hand, are ineligible for all publicly funded services besides perinatal and emergency room care. However, this generally precludes comprehensive care and can be financially untenable. The cumulative effects of social disadvantage are well established and suggest that "the costliest consequences of unauthorized status will emerge later in the life course, as current generations of unauthorized parents, children, and youth move into midlife and older age" (Suárez-Orozco et al. 2011: 457). With an estimated 4.5 million US citizen children living in mixed-status families, along with an additional one million undocumented children, a lack of access to medical care deters the integration of communities and relegates even citizens to a second-class social status (O'Leary and Sanchez 2011).

As a result of having members with different legal statuses, these families experience a number of different opportunities and restrictions on accessing healthcare. This impacts the social mobility and well-being of the entire family. Parents in mixed-status families must cultivate the ability to seek healthcare in multiple sites, with distinct plans for individual members, depending on their status (Castañeda and Melo 2014). Thus, insured individuals, including US-born children with Medicaid, are able to visit private physicians' practices and urgent care clinics, while undocumented and/or uninsured individuals must avoid getting sick. When they do, they can be seen at one of the community health centers that operate on a sliding-scale basis (that is, with flexible fees depending on income) or by one of the limited charity clinics in the region.

When siblings with different forms of access become ill at the same time, as is often the case with colds and other common childhood infections, mothers can spend the greater part of a day or two first visiting a pediatrician for the child with Medicaid, followed by long waits at charity or community clinics hoping to have an undocumented child seen for the same condition. This results in time off from work and loss of income and is logistically difficult if no transportation is available. In this largely rural area, there are no buses or taxis, and transportation can be a huge hurdle for the very poor. Veronica has lived in the United States for eight years, having moved here with her husband. She is a thirty-four-year-old mother of five children with different statuses: three are US citizens, and two were born in Mexico and are currently undocumented. Veronica described the journey that an episode of illness provokes:

> Well, for the ones with Medicaid, I call their doctor. If they are very sick, they even try to see them the same day I call. But for the older two, if

> one of them has a fever that won't end, I have to take him to [the charity clinic]. They are only open certain hours and there is always a line. If my husband is working, I don't have a car and then I have to ask a neighbor to take us. It's a lot.[1]

In another example, Jonathan, a twenty-two-year-old undocumented college student who grew up with two US citizen brothers, talks about the added barriers and costs uninsured family members face, including the unwillingness to call an ambulance:

> I just knew that when my little brothers would need dental care, healthcare, they would qualify for that because of Medicaid. So they were lucky enough for that, but my parents and me, it was a different story. We would get sick and look for remedies at home, or if we had to, would go to the health center, or other times when I would get sick, I would have to go to the hospital, so the bills were always so high. You had to avoid going anywhere.

Restricted Mobility and Travel for Specialty Care

As noted earlier, those with unauthorized or unclear legal status are unable to travel to other parts of the state, as this requires inspection at CBP checkpoints along all highways. These permanent, tollbooth-like checkpoints are a fact of life along the US–Mexico border, stretching along all lanes of major highways that lead into the interior of the United States, visible from many miles away and impossible to avoid. They are located not at the actual border (where there are separate and much more thorough inspections), but approximately seventy miles inland. As motorists approach, cones corral their vehicles, organizing them into lanes. Agents and drug-sniffing dogs stand at the ready to inspect all vehicles. Checkpoints have increased in recent years and have drawn the ire of many residents, with US citizens—also subject to inspection—arguing that this violates their constitutional right against arbitrary stops and searches (Santos 2014) and illustrating well the racial and ethnic profiling that border communities are subjected to on a daily basis.

Several participants thus described feeling "trapped" or "stuck" by these geophysical limitations—the militarized US–Mexico border on one side, and the US border patrol checkpoints on the other—and many had not left the Rio Grande Valley in decades. Nonetheless, people sometimes needed to cross a checkpoint in order to seek out specialized medical care. Some families reported an inability to travel to specialized schools (for children who are blind or deaf, for instance, the closest schools are located in major cities beyond the checkpoints) or to access tertiary care (e.g., cancer treatments or severe burn care).

In addition, people have experienced difficulties accompanying family members—including their own minor children—if specialists are located in major cities beyond the checkpoints. A community health center physician relayed the story of an eight-year-old girl diagnosed with leukemia the year before. The only treatment available for her complex pediatric case was at MD Anderson Cancer Center in Houston, which lies on the other side of the border patrol checkpoints on US Highway 281 (or, alternatively, US-77). Although the girl was a US citizen and her care covered through Medicaid, her mother was undocumented. Even a copy of the girl's medical records with the diagnosis and a letter from the physician addressed to CBP did not suffice to permit the mother to cross into the interior of the state. There was no guarantee that the mother would not be deported if she approached the checkpoint with her child. In anguish, "she had to put her daughter on a Greyhound bus, with her fourteen-year-old brother as the guardian" accompanying her on the trip to Houston, according to the physician. "It's just immoral," he said, "for us as a society to expect a mother to stay behind while her eight-year-old daughter has to travel four hundred miles away for treatment. To tell her, 'No, you're not allowed to go'. In what world is that all right?"

Cross-Border Care

In recent years, alternative and informal channels of care have been proliferating because formal systems have been largely unable meet the needs of a large segment of the population. Primary among these is crossing the border to visit medical professionals or to buy medications in Mexico. Elvia, a fifty-five-year-old legal permanent resident who has lived in the United States for almost twenty years, still travels to Mexico regularly to see her family physician in Reynosa, just on the other side of the river. She says,

> I go whenever I need to. Like recently, I was undergoing menopause [*tuve el cambio de vida*] and having heavy bleeding. I went to my doctor in Mexico because the doctors here wouldn't give me anything, no pill, nothing. They would do blood tests, tell me I was anemic, but give me nothing. The one time they did give me something, it was too expensive. It is so much cheaper to buy it over there. So I went to my doctor over there and she gave me a shot that made it stop. And medications that I could afford.

In addition to their affordability, Mexican medicines are described by many people as "better" because they are "stronger" or "the full dose," as opposed to what is prescribed in the United States. As others have shown

(Horton and Cole 2011), medical returns to Mexico are common even among Latinos who do have health insurance—like Elvia—because of the distinct culture of medicine as practiced in these border clinics, leading to higher patient satisfaction.

However, increased border policing has reduced the ability to cross back and forth for medical care or medications, since those with uncertain legal status face more scrutiny of their documents than ever before. As a result, fewer people are crossing the border to Mexico for medical and dental services—something that was common in previous years. In addition, many legal permanent residents and US citizens now hesitate to access care across the border because of the cartel violence in the neighboring Mexican state of Tamaulipas. Simultaneously, many health professionals have relocated their practices farther into the interior of Mexico to avoid extortion fees demanded by cartels. The irony here, for undocumented persons, is that even as Mexican citizens they are no longer able to obtain medical care there because they would be unable to return to their home in the United States. Thus, they face restricted mobility—literally—in both directions.

Mobile Medicines and Mobile Providers

Regional geography and heavy law enforcement presence impact healthcare-seeking experiences in unique ways. This region has a vast informal economy, fostered by the international border, high poverty, and inequality (Richardson and Pisani 2012). In some cases, the mobility of medicines is the result of US citizens or permanent residents accessing resources in Mexico. In addition, some Mexican citizens can apply for a Border Crossing Card (often referred to as a "laser visa," a B1/B2 visitor's visa issued for ten years at a time) that allows them to cross back and forth on a regular basis. This visa recognizes the interdependence of border communities, as people cross frequently to work and spend time with relatives. To qualify, applicants must demonstrate sufficient business, employment, family, or property ties in Mexico. While holders are not permitted to reside in the United States, this visa does allow frequent, short-term transnational opportunities.

Medicines from Mexico

A result of increased enforcement and an inability to travel to Mexico for care is reliance on family members with greater ability to cross the border, whether Mexican or American. Increasingly, rather than crossing the border themselves, people will ask or pay others to do so. For instance, Elvia, the fifty-five-year-old legal permanent resident introduced earlier, described bringing back medications from Mexico for her two undocumented teenage grandsons:

> Like with the flu or something, well, I just bring them medicines over from Mexico. I go to the doctor I have there, the one we always consult over there, and tell him, 'they have this, this, and that' and he will just write me a prescription. The medicines are much cheaper over there.

There has also been an increase in strategies such as purchasing prescription medications that are offered—unlawfully and in an unregulated manner—by vendors at local flea markets, especially antibiotics, steroids to treat inflammation, insulin for diabetes, weight-loss medicines, and birth control pills.

As women's health services have been increasingly defunded in Texas over the past several years—restricting access to abortion but also to the few locations where uninsured women could access *any* healthcare—emergency contraception has been in high demand in informal markets, particularly a small, white, hexagonal pill called misoprostol. Also known as miso or Cytotec (*cytoteca* in Spanish), the drug induces a miscarriage-like abortion during the early stages of a pregnancy. In the Rio Grande Valley, both abortion clinics were closed in the wake of efforts by the Republican-led state legislature. In 2013, House Bill 2 (HB2) required clinics with abortion care to have hospital-like facilities, including a prescribed minimum width of hallways and doorways, piping for anesthesia, and admitting privileges for clinic physicians at a hospital within 30 miles. Following the closures, the closest clinic for women living in the Rio Grande Valley was 150 miles away—and, notably, on the other side of the checkpoint (Hellerstein 2014). For many poor women in the region, that distance is beyond feasible, especially given the transportation limitations described earlier. For undocumented women, crossing the checkpoint would be impossible anyway. Opponents appealed the laws, and in 2016, the US Supreme Court struck down HB2. While some abortion care clinics in the state were able to reopen, only one has begun offering abortion services in the Rio Grande Valley again (Fleuriet and Castañeda 2017).

Sharing Medicines

Another way in which medicines themselves become "mobile" is through the sharing of prescription medications. It is not uncommon for medicines prescribed to a US citizen child, who has access to insurance and other programs, to also be used to treat undocumented siblings or parents. Jonathan, the twenty-two-year-old undocumented college student introduced earlier, described how commonplace this practice is:

> Let's say you get a cold or something. Yeah, we [he and his parents] would get sick too, but we would use medicines from, like, when people prescribed something to my brothers [who had Medicaid]. They didn't use all of them, so we would use them. That is how we would do it.

The circulation of "leftover" medication takes place both within a family as well as in the broader community through social ties, as Angela, a nineteen-year-old US citizen with undocumented parents, illustrates: "My mom has diabetes. Usually she has friends who have, like, leftover insulin or stuff like that. They just give it to her."

Medication practices are socially embedded phenomena, and saving, sharing, and reusing them is common in most marginal communities. Sharing medications not only serves the immediate need of treating illness but also acts as an important resource in settings where medical care and affordable medications may be scarce. It creates the social obligation of reciprocity within a family and within a community, offering a reserve resource for people to call upon in times of need. However, it is not without risk: a diabetic using insulin requires regular medical attention to ensure proper dosage (which may change over time), and in the case of shared antibiotics—by far the most widely circulated medicine—failure to complete the full prescribed dose may lead to the emergence of drug-resistant pathogens.

Informal Providers

The vast health inequalities in the region, coupled with a decreased ability to travel to Mexico, have created an even more lucrative market for informal healthcare providers practicing without a license. In some cases, unlicensed practitioners operate out of their own homes or at flea markets (Castañeda 2016). These are typically dentists licensed in Mexico but not in the United States, or nursing assistants who provide injections for a fee (although not legally permitted to do so).

Some dentists operate out of their own homes or will make house calls to patients' homes. Marina, a forty-two-year-old woman, described the situation in the following way:

> There are no dentists here for us. Some come from Mexico and we seek them out in homes, but it is risky for them because they could get caught, could get in trouble. But we need them. My mother has gone to such dentists who are not licensed here. I need to go, too, but I am afraid. It's not the same, like being in a clinic where you know exactly how everything was cleaned, and that they have everything they need. To work out of a house, it could be that they have cleaned everything, but it's better not to do it that way.

Increasingly strict border enforcement in recent years has produced many of these informal practices, which are in part related to an inability to travel for affordable medical care in Mexico. With limited opportunities to obtain services, many residents in the US–Mexico borderlands are forced to seek healthcare that is improvisational and may pose additional risks to their health.

Conclusion

This chapter has examined the contradictory processes by which mobility associated with healthcare access and delivery is both fostered and hindered in communities along the US–Mexico border. In the case described here, particular groups experience a "stuckness" (Cresswell 2012), in which their movement is constrained by a stillness produced and imposed through larger bordering processes. A rethinking of borders as dynamic and inhabited places—as "borderscapes," perhaps (dell'Agnese and Szary 2015)—allows us to shift our focus from the stillness of the border fence or wall to the stillness or stuckness of people, such as those described in this chapter.

Here, I have shown how this stuckness has powerful impacts on the ability of some people to access healthcare services. This issue has received increased attention in recent years, since border communities account for the largest percentage of the uninsured population and continue to be classified as medically underserved areas. Achieving health equity in the United States will be impossible without addressing the needs of these communities. One way of understanding their marginality is through the lens of "deservingness"—that is, the ways in which some groups but not others are considered worthy of health-related attention, investment, and care (Willen 2012)—and thus linked to larger questions of inequality and the interconnectedness of multiple systems of entitlement. Distinct from formalized entitlements and pragmatic questions of access, this allows us to understand the subtler moral positions that undergird both in a scenario where immigration and healthcare policy are intertwined, and where securitization discourse supersedes the health needs of otherwise vibrant communities. The borderlands context includes extreme poverty, deprivation, and intense everyday surveillance, but also resilience and creativity, as evidenced by the practices described here. The people living between the international border and the checkpoints that prevent them from entering the nation's interior are people who have become "stuck in motion," experiencing simultaneous mobility and immobility.

Acknowledgments

Funding for this research was provided by the National Science Foundation and the Wenner-Gren Foundation for Anthropological Research. I would like to thank Milena A. Melo for her invaluable assistance on the project, particularly with recruitment and data collection, and Nora Brickhouse Arriola, Carla Castillo, Ryan Logan, and Aria Walsh-Felz for their assistance with transcription and analysis.

Heide Castañeda, PhD, is an associate professor in the Department of Anthropology at the University of South Florida. Her research focuses on health inequalities related to unauthorized migration, especially the analysis of legal status and constructs of citizenship. She is author of *Borders of Belonging: Struggle and Solidarity in Mixed-Status Immigrant Families* (Stanford University Press, 2019). Her work has appeared in *Unequal Coverage: The Experience of Health Care Reform in the United States* (New York University Press, 2017) and *Living Together, Living Apart: Mixed Status Families and US Immigration Policy* (University of Washington Press, 2015), as well as in journals including *Social Science & Medicine*, *Journal of Health Care for the Poor and Underserved*, *Annual Review of Public Health*, and *American Ethnologist*.

NOTE

1. All quotes have been translated by the author into English from the original Spanish.

REFERENCES

Abrego, Leisy J., and Cecilia Menjívar. 2011. "Immigrant Latina Mothers as Targets of Legal Violence." *International Journal of Sociology of the Family* 37(1): 9–26.

Bastida, Elena, H. Shelton Brown III, and José A. Pagán. 2008. "Persistent Disparities in the Use of Health Care along the US-Mexico Border: An Ecological Perspective." *American Journal of Public Health* 98(11): 1987–95.

Blunt, Alison. 2007. "Cultural Geographies of Migration: Mobility, Transnationality, and Diaspora." *Progress in Human Geography* 31(5): 684–94.

Capps, Randolph, Michael E. Fix, Jason Ost, Jane Reardon-Anderson, and Jeffrey S. Passel. 2004. *The Health and Well-Being of Young Children of Immigrants*. Washington, DC: The Urban Institute.

Castañeda, Heide. 2016. "Health Care along the U.S./Mexico Border." In *The Routledge Handbook of Medical Anthropology*, ed. Lenore Manderson, Anita Hardon, and Elizabeth Cartwright, 269–273. New York: Routledge.

——. 2017a. "Is Coverage Enough? Persistent Health Disparities in Marginalized Latino Border Communities." *Journal of Ethnic and Migration Studies* 43(12): 2003–19.

——. 2017b. "Stratification by Immigration Status: Contradictory Exclusion and Inclusion after Health Care Reform." In *Unequal Coverage: The Experience of Health Care Reform in the United States,* ed. Jessica Mulligan and Heide Castañeda, 37–58. New York: New York University Press.

Castañeda, Heide, and Milena A. Melo. 2014. "Health Care Access for Latino Mixed-Status Families: Barriers, Strategies, and Implications for Reform." *American Behavioral Scientist* 58(14): 1891–909.

Castañeda, Heide, Seth M. Holmes, Daniel S. Madrigal, Maria-Elena DeTrinidad Young, Naomi Beyerle, and James Quesada. 2015. "Immigration as a Social Determinant of Health." *Annual Review of Public Health* 36: 375–92.

Cresswell, Tim. 2006. "The Right to Mobility: The Production of Mobility in the Courtroom." *Antipode* 38(4): 735–54.

——. 2012. "Mobilities II: Still." *Progress in Human Geography* 36: 645–53.

dell'Agnese, Elena, and Anne-Laure Amilhat Szary. 2015. "Borderscapes: From Border Landscapes to Border Aesthetics." *Geopolitics* 20(1): 4–13.

Fleuriet, K. Jill, and Heide Castañeda. 2017. "A Risky Place? Media and the Health Landscape in the (In)secure U.S.-Mexico Borderlands." *North American Dialogue* 20(2): 32–46.

Gonzales, Roberto G. 2011. "Learning to Be Illegal: Undocumented Youth and Shifting Legal Contexts in the Transition to Adulthood." *American Sociological Review* 76(4): 602–19.

Hagan, Jacqueline, Nestor Rodriguez, Randy Capps, and Nika Kabiri. 2003. "The Effects of Recent Welfare and Immigration Reforms on Immigrants' Access to Health Care." *International Migration Review* 37(2): 444–63.

Hannam, Kevin, Mimi Sheller, and John Urry. 2006. "Editorial: Mobilities, Immobilities and Moorings." *Mobilities* 1(1): 1–22.

Hellerstein, Erica. 2014. "The Rise of the DYI Abortion in Texas." *The Atlantic,* 27 June.

Heyman, Josiah McC. 2008. "Constructing a Virtual Wall: Race and Citizenship in U.S.-Mexico Border Policing." *Journal of the Southwest* 50(3): 305–33.

——. 2010. "The State and Mobile People at the U.S.-Mexico Border." In *Class, Contention, and a World in Motion,* ed. Winnie Lem and Pauline Gardiner Barber, 58–78. New York: Berghahn Books.

Horton, Sarah, and Stephanie Cole. 2011. "Medical Returns: Seeking Health Care in Mexico." *Social Science & Medicine* 72(11): 1846–52.

Huang, Zhihuan Jennifer, Stella M. Yu, and Rebecca Ledsky. 2006. "Health Status and Health Service Access and Use among Children in U.S. Immigrant Families." *American Journal of Public Health* 96(4): 634–40.

Mangual Figueroa, Ariana M. 2012. "'I Have Papers So I Can Go Anywhere!': Everyday Talk about Citizenship in a Mixed-Status Mexican Family." *Journal of Language, Identity & Education* 11(5): 291–311.

Mendoza, Fernando S. 2009. "Health Disparities and Children in Immigrant Families: A Research Agenda." *Pediatrics* 124(S3): S187–95.

Menjívar, Cecilia, and Leisy Abrego. 2009. "Parents and Children across Borders: Legal Instability and Intergenerational Relations in Guatemalan and Salvadoran Families." In *Across Generations: Immigrant Families in America,* ed. N. Foner, 160–189. New York: New York University Press.

Mier, Nelda, Isadore Flores, John R. C. Robinson, and Ann V. Millard. 2004. "Cultural, Demographic, Educational, and Economic Characteristics." In *Nourishing the Future: The Case for Community-Based Nutrition Research in the Lower Rio Grande Valley,* ed. R. S. Day, 15–24. Houston, TX: University of Texas School of Public Health at Houston.

O'Leary, Anna Ochoa., and Azucena Sanchez. 2011. "Anti-immigrant Arizona: Ripple Effects and Mixed Immigration Status Households under 'Policies of Attrition' Considered." *Journal of Borderlands Studies* 4(26): 115–33.

Park, Lisa S. 2011. "Criminalizing Immigrant Mothers: Public Charge, Health Care, and Welfare Reform." *International Journal of Sociology of the Family* 37(1): 27–47.

Passel, Jeffrey S. 2011. "Demography of Immigrant Youth: Past, Present, Future." *Future of Children* 21(1): 19–41.

Pereira, Krista M., Robert Crosnoe, Karina Fortuny, Juan Pedroza, Kjertsi Ulvestad, Christina Weiland, Hirokazu Yoshikawa, and Ajay Chaudry. 2012. *Barriers to Immigrants' Access to Health and Human Services Programs.* Retrieved from http://aspe.hhs.gov/hsp/11/ImmigrantAccess/Barriers/rb.pdf.

Richardson, Chad, and Michael J. Pisani. 2012. *The Informal and Underground Economy of the South Texas Border.* Austin, TX: University of Texas Press.

Salazar, Noel B., Alice Elliot, and Roger Norum. 2017. "Studying Mobilities: Theoretical Notes and Methodological Queries." In *Methodologies of Mobility: Ethnography and Experiment,* ed. Alice Elliot, Roger Norum, and Noel B. Salazar, 1–24. Oxford, UK: Berghahn Books.

Santos, Fernanda. 2014. "Border Patrol Scrutiny Stirs Anger in Arizona Town." *New York Times,* 28 June, A13.

Sheller, Mimi, and John Urry. 2006. "The New Mobilities Paradigm." *Environment and Planning A* 38(2): 207–26.

Sommers, Benjamin D. 2013. "Stuck between Health and Immigration Reform—Care for Undocumented Immigrants." *New England Journal of Medicine* 369: 593–95.

Stuesse, Angela, and Mathew Coleman. 2014. "Automobility, Immobility, Altermobility: Surviving and Resisting the Intensification of Immigrant Policing." *City & Society* 26(1): 51–72.

Suárez-Orozco, Carolina, Hirokazu Yoshikawa, Robert T. Teranishi, and Marcelo M. Suárez-Orozco. 2011. "Growing Up in the Shadows: The Developmental Implications of Unauthorized Status." *Harvard Educational Review* 81(3): 438–73.

Willen, Sarah S. 2012. "Migration, 'Illegality,' and Health: Mapping Embodied Vulnerability and Debating Health-Related Deservingness." *Social Science & Medicine* 74(6): 805–11.

Willen, Sarah S., Jessica Mulligan, and Heide Castañeda. 2011. "Take a Stand Commentary: How Can Medical Anthropologists Contribute to Contemporary Conversations on 'Illegal' Im/migration and Health?" *Medical Anthropology Quarterly* 25(3): 331–56.

Winton, Ailsa. 2015. "Violence, Borders, and Boundaries: Reframing Young People's Mobility." In *Movement, Mobilities, and Journeys: Geographies of Children and Young People*, ed. C.N. Laoire, A. White, and T. Skelton, 1–19. Singapore: Springer.

Xu, Qingwen, and Kalina Brabeck. 2012. "Service Utilization for Latino Children in Mixed-Status Families." *Social Work Research* 36(3): 209–21.

CHAPTER 2

"It's Too Risky to Leave the House"

Immigrant Policing and Health-Related Mobility

Nolan Kline

Unlike most people her age living in Atlanta, Georgia, Sarita, an undocumented woman in her early twenties, will not drive a car in her suburban neighborhood. She could easily pass a Georgia state driver's license test, and she works enough hours that she could save money to purchase a car. Sarita is not afraid to be behind the wheel of a vehicle, and she knows the roadways in her Atlanta neighborhood well, as is evident at our first meeting. When I arrived at Sarita's house for the interview we scheduled, she jumped into the car, shaking her hair still wet from the shower. "Can we stop at Walmart?" Sarita asked. "Sure," my research collaborator, who was driving, replied, taking us a few miles down the road to the mega retailer chain. When we arrived, we all exited the car and my collaborator and I were confused about why we had made a detour to the retail warehouse, with its hazy lighting bouncing off a worn, white floor. Once in the store, Sarita went to a photo station with a disposable camera in hand. While we waited for her photos to be developed, she told us about a rally she and other undocumented youth had hosted recently. "I want to show you the pictures, and once they're done we can go somewhere to talk."

After a blue-vested cashier took Sarita's money, we piled back into the car and began our journey to a local library, where we would secure a room to talk about Sarita's experience as an undocumented youth activist. Along the way, Sarita pointed out where local police would set up roadblocks and ask for driver's licenses of Latinx-looking motorists.[1] "That corner is really bad, especially at night. . . . The police come out way more at night, so I had to change jobs." Sarita works as a server at a restaurant near her home. Even though she sometimes works a late shift, requiring her to leave as late as 3:00 AM on some nights, Sarita is grateful she can get to her job without having to drive. As she explained to me in the car, she and her family do not leave the house in a car at night when police are more likely to be in her neighborhood "We don't leave the house after 10:00 PM because there are too many police around. It doesn't matter if you're sick, if you need medicine—nothing. It's too risky to leave the house."

Sarita and her family's cautious efforts to limit their driving and avoid police reflects overall changes in some undocumented Latinx immigrants' mobility as a response to harsh immigrant-policing regimes. In particular, Sarita's statement about not leaving the house even in situations of medical need illustrates how changing mobility patterns can directly impact some immigrants' health. Not leaving the house at certain times of day is not the only way in which immigration enforcement has impacted undocumented immigrants in Atlanta, however. The complex web of enforcement has resulted in numerous health-related mobility changes for several undocumented Latinxs I met. This chapter demonstrates how immigrant policing—the confluence of multiple immigration laws and police practices that merge and increase undocumented immigrants' risk of deportation (Kline 2017)—operates in ways that directly shape undocumented Latinx immigrants' health-related mobility.

In focusing on mobility and health, I build upon Vindrola-Padros, Johnson, and Pfister (this volume), who argue that movement and stasis can be a "window into social constructions of gender, class, ability, ethnicity" and other ways of living in the world that also shape how health services are obtained and delivered. Moreover, the concept of mobility is important in health and social science research since mobility can be both a barrier to accessing health services and an enabling factor in receiving care. Limited mobility, for example, can hinder access to health services, and among some populations, such as migrant farmworkers, a highly mobile lifestyle is one of many hindrances in receiving healthcare (Wilson et al. 2000; Weathers et al. 2003; Gwyther and Jenkins 1998). Mobility related to health services is therefore often conceived as a determinant that lies within a spectrum shaping health; too much mobility hinders healthcare, and not enough mobility impedes access to services. Rather than focusing on mobility as a health determinant, however, I examine the determinants of mobility itself, which are linked to broader social phenomena and driven by specific political agendas. As the experiences of immigrants and service providers in this chapter highlight, immigrant policing has altered the forms of mobility that have shaped both healthcare access and preferred forms of healthcare delivery for many of the undocumented immigrants I met in Atlanta.

Methods

During one year of ethnographic fieldwork in Atlanta, between June 2012 and June 2013, I examined how immigration enforcement impacted immigrants' health and the communities in which they live. Atlanta is home to a new Latinx immigrant population that grew rapidly between 2000 and 2010. Since 2010, Georgia has passed several aggressive immigration laws, prompting responses from immigrant rights groups. As a medical anthropologist embracing an activist research perspective (Hale 2006; Pulido 2008), I worked closely with immigrant rights organizations during my fieldwork, where I met undocumented immigrants who were willing to share their experiences with me. In addition to embracing an activist-oriented form of ethnography, I also aimed to trace the connections of immigrant policing through multiple social spaces, leading me to adopt a multisited ethnographic methodology.

Multisited ethnography is a form of fieldwork where the researcher examines a specific topic through multiple social spaces (Marcus 1995). As a form of ethnography dedicated to understanding pathways and threads of ideas and social phenomena, multisited ethnography is a way of responding to challenges in mobilities research, such as understanding how social processes take on different forms in different places (Büscher and Urry 2009). In adopting a multisited approach, I interviewed immigrants, leaders of health-related nongovernmental organizations, policymakers, immigrant rights leaders, physicians, and hospital administrators. These data-collection activities gave me insight into how immigrant policing impacts immigrants' lives and the communities in which they live. Conducting multisited research demanded that I adopt a mobile research paradigm (Sheller and Urry 2006) and occasionally engage in what felt to me like "ethnography on the go," traveling between immigrant rights organizations, the Georgia state capitol, hospitals, immigrants' homes, and a variety of other locations. In engaging in a form of "mobile ethnography" and staying attentive to my privilege as a researcher, I conducted interviews with undocumented immigrants in places of their choice, mostly in their homes, to reduce their risk of encountering a harsh immigration regime. To protect participants' identities, all individuals and organizations named in this chapter have been assigned pseudonyms.

Immigrant Policing in the United States

In numerous parts of the United States, undocumented immigrants like Sarita are under near-constant threat of being detected by police, arrested, and deported. The threat of deportation stems from aggressive state and federal immigration laws that combine with local police practices to exacerbate undocumented immigrants' vulnerability to having their immigration status discovered. These layered immigrant-policing efforts make mundane spaces such as local roadways potential sites of danger, as local law enforcement agents become de facto immigration officers (Menjívar 2014; Coleman 2012). The potential for deportation is especially acute in states like Georgia, a state that implemented an aggressive local immigrant-policing law: the Illegal Immigration Reform and Enforcement Act of 2011, or House Bill (HB) 87. Modeled after other aggressive immigration legislation in Arizona, HB 87 extends federal immigration powers to local police by allowing officers to stop, detain, and arrest any person suspected of being undocumented. Once an officer stops a driver suspected of being undocumented, or a driver with passengers suspected of being undocumented, the law enforcement agent asks for a driver's license from the suspected undocumented immigrant. Since undocumented immigrants are banned from obtaining driver's licenses in Georgia, an undocumented driver or passenger is unable to produce one. The officer can then arrest an immigrant driver or passenger for not having a driver's license; impound the driver's vehicle, which they must sometimes pay a large fee to retrieve; and place any children in the car in custody with someone else. Once the arrestee is taken to jail, his or her fingerprints are taken and assessed through a federal database as part of the United States' Secure Communities program.

Secure Communities is one of the most robust federal immigration efforts. Through the program, fingerprints taken at local jailhouses are compared with existing records for possible criminal infractions and immigration concerns. If no fingerprint match is found, or if a found match indicates an unauthorized immigration status, an automatic Immigration and Customs Enforcement (ICE) hold is placed on the arrestee for three days until an ICE agent can come and verify the detainee's status. Another federal program, section 287(g) of the Immigration and Nationality Act, deputizes local law enforcement as federal agents, granting them federal authority to enforce immigration statutes. In Georgia, four counties participate in the 287(g) program, three of which are in the Atlanta metropolitan area. In the aggregate, immigrant-policing initiatives comprising state and federal statutes and local police practices creates mobility challenges for undocumented immigrants in Atlanta. Through immigrant-policing regimes, the act of driving or being an undocumented passenger in a car becomes a high-risk activity that can result in forced removal from the United States and family separation.

Aggressive immigrant-policing efforts in the United States are designed to use law enforcement in a way to encourage immigrants to "self-deport" based on an "attrition through enforcement" strategy (Su 2012; Kobach 2008). These policies not only impact immigrant communities, but also affect nonimmigrant populations. For example, Georgia's HB 87 initially criminalized any type of assistance provided to undocumented immigrants, implicating taxicab drivers, clergy, and healthcare workers providing nonemergency care as lawbreakers. The breadth of laws like HB 87 points to how such policies aim both to impact undocumented immigrants' lives and to destabilize any type of support they receive. Furthermore, as a way of disrupting immigrants' lives, immigrant-policing efforts have had negative consequences on immigrants' family relationships, creating stress among parents about being separated from their children and anxiety among children who worry about their parents being deported (White et al. 2014; Dreby 2012; Allen, Cisneros, and Tellez 2015). Similarly, immigrant policing can be detrimental to immigrants' individual health behaviors, making immigrants more fearful of seeking specific types of health services (Hardy et al. 2012; Hacker et al. 2011; Rhodes et al. 2015; Alexander and Fernandez 2014; Kline 2017).

Immigrant-policing initiatives contribute to undocumented immigrants' overall health-related structural vulnerabilities. As an analytical lens attentive to how social processes shape experiences, structural vulnerability emphasizes how undocumented status, or "illegality," shapes immigrants' potential for economic exploitation, racial discrimination, and, generally, perceptions of needing punishment and being undeserving of social services (Quesada, Hart, and Bourgois 2011). Policy, including immigration-enforcement laws and police practices, contributes to undocumented immigrants' structural vulnerability and specifically transforms immigrants' mobility, shaping their overall healthcare experiences and reshaping their preferred healthcare delivery methods.

(Auto)mobility and Health

Mobility encompasses a broad range of social and biological phenomena and is directly linked to health experiences and outcomes. The term can refer to physical capabilities, activities, movement, geographic contexts, and social factors impacting life chances to move through socioeconomic levels (for examples, see Cardano, Costa, and Demaria 2004; Dahl 1996; Mao et al. 2015; Wullems et al. 2016). Furthermore, since mobility is linked to historical and political contexts, it is an especially useful concept in examining social concerns for undocumented immigrants in the United States, whose social and political mobilities are often questioned because of their immigration status and articulated "undeservingness" of receiving publicly funded health services (Sullivan and Rehm 2005; Zapata Roblyer et al. 2015; Alcántara, Chen, and Alegría 2014). More directly, mobility can affect undocumented immigrants' access to health services and may impact physical and mental health. Beyond being a variable that is linked to health status, mobility is also an important theoretical tool for examining how social phenomena like immigrant policing work to indirectly impact immigrants' overall well-being.

Rather than focusing on physical capabilities or socioeconomic mobility, I examine mobility through geographic space, primarily through the use of automobiles—the way in which the majority of US residents navigate both urban and rural landscapes. Automobiles and driving are an especially important aspect of mobility in the United States because they are integral to important activities. The majority of US residents get to work by using an automobile, and US residents use the highly developed automobile-specific infrastructure to drive to health clinics, grocery stores, and pharmacies, and to reach any location needed for maintaining their overall health and well-being. Moreover, because automobiles are a central component of life in the United States, use of automobiles is highly regulated and automobile safety is a public health priority. For undocumented immigrants in the United States, aggressive immigration laws alter the relationship between health and automobile-specific mobility.

Social scientists have drawn attention to how severe immigration regimes impact immigrants' mobility and, specifically, restrict their mobility by creating challenges and risks associated with driving (Amuedo-Dorantes, Puttitanun, and Martinez-Donate 2013). More than a mode of transportation, cars involve a range of emotional responses and include elements of political regulation and safety assessments (Sheller 2004). They are important fixtures in modern urban geography, allowing for sprawl in major metropolitan areas like Atlanta, and cars play a critical role in how space is organized and planned (Böhm et al. 2006; Sheller and Urry 2000). Furthermore, cars, driving, and the infrastructure dedicated to automobiles play an important role in social organization and social experiences. Accordingly, the analytical frame of "automobility" captures the complexities of cars and their broader social significance.

The term "automobility" refers to numerous ideas related to cars and movement, including industrial production and Fordism, consumption, social and technical assemblages linked to cars (like roadside assistance services and motels), private types of mobility and their status in relationship to public mobility, and environmental relationships between people and their products (Beckmann 2001). More simply, automobility can describe how people use automobiles and their associated infrastructure to live their lives in particular ways (Beckmann 2001; Cresswell 2006, 2010; Sheller 2004; Sheller and Urry 2000). Since cars and the infrastructure associated with them are key elements of life, focusing on automobility provides a way to examine how lives can be changed or interrupted by social phenomena such as police practices and localized enforcement of immigration laws.

Exploring immigrant policing through the lens of automobility, Stuesse and Coleman (2014) demonstrate how immigrant-policing initiatives largely leave undocumented immigrants in a state of compromised mobility whereby navigating urban spaces is associated with risk of deportation. Roadways, designed to facilitate individual mobility, thus become risky spaces and encourage immobility for undocumented immigrants. Borrowing from theories of biopolitics—the way in which power is applied over all aspects of life (Foucault 2003)—I aimed to understand how immigrant policing is a type of political power that shapes immigrants' health. Ultimately, I found that policing affects undocumented immigrants' health by shaping their automobility.

Changing Health-Related Mobility

Limiting Exposure to Police

As a result of increasingly harsh immigrant-policing regimes, some undocumented immigrants in Atlanta changed their health-related mobility in ways similar to those of Sarita and her family. Just as Sarita described avoiding leaving the house at certain times of day even if someone was sick, other immigrants reported not driving in certain areas because they knew police would be nearby. One woman, Griselda, for example, lived in an apartment complex near an intersection where police routinely set up checkpoints. Griselda moved to Atlanta from Mexico in 2005, leaving behind her four-month-old daughter in search of better economic opportunities. In Atlanta, she routinely drove to work—an activity she knew was risky but was necessary in order to get to her job. "I didn't use to drive, but driving is a necessity to get to work. . . . You have to be able to drive yourself. I drive, but until now, thank God, a police officer has never stopped me or anything." Griselda has been fortunate to have never been stopped by police, and for this she credits strategically avoiding roadblocks and reducing the times she drives. "There are areas that, for example, we know where they put up roadblocks, and it's better to not go through there or keep going—more at night or in the afternoon they put up the roadblocks." Because she drives in the morning and early evening, Griselda has been able to avoid the roadblocks and thus avoid deportation. "They put up the roadblocks by Latino business because they know there are many Hispanics or a lot of Latinos that go by there," she added. "So now you drive with fear because sometimes you know the police can stop you."

These feelings of fear that Griselda described tended to influence where some undocumented immigrants would seek health services. Some immigrants I met in Atlanta would seek care in places that were easily accessible to them, minimizing their driving time and thereby minimizing their potential exposure to police and risk of arrest. For many immigrants, "safe" spaces for health services included informal providers who operated out of their garages, on their patios, or in their living rooms; traditional folk healers; pharmacies that sold prescription medication over the counter; and "Latinx clinics": small, fee-for-service clinics that advertise to Latinxs and have Spanish-speaking staff. These spaces were seen as free from the threat of deportation, and Latinx clinics, in particular, were successful in attracting undocumented patients because they offered a variety of services on a fee-for-service basis and were seen as safe locations. As one leader of a health organization for Latinx immigrants explained, "a lot of these [Latinx] clinics are really successful: they offer prenatal care, they offer physicals, checkups, all of that, and people know, and they trust that they're not going to be deported if they go there and are undocumented." Although some undocumented immigrants and health organization leaders expressed suspicion over the quality of these clinics, they nevertheless noted that Latinx clinics are typically in Latinx neighborhoods and therefore reduce the risk of encountering police while driving. Seeking care at Latinx clinics has thus become a risk-mitigating option for undocumented Latinx immigrants in Atlanta.

While informal or Latinx clinics were viable options for some undocumented immigrants' care, seeking services at a hospital or large clinic was sometimes necessary since not all Latinx clinics or informal providers could treat all of their patients' health concerns. Needing more advanced forms of treatment but still fearing exposure to police, some undocumented immigrants would take taxis or pay friends for rides to healthcare settings, adding to the overall cost of care. For example, Jimena, a nurse at a health department in the Atlanta area explained that after immigrant-policing efforts intensified, she saw more patients taking taxis to the clinic out of necessity. "If they don't have somebody to bring them, or no means of transportation, they take a taxi . . . so if you don't have the money for a taxi you're not going to come." The Latinx patients Jimena sees have restricted financial means, and the need to take a taxi exacerbates the financial burden of healthcare. "And then if they need to come back . . . so every time it's a taxi, and it's expensive, and a lot of people don't want to drive because they don't have a license and they think they're going to get pulled over, and if they get pulled over [the police] are going to take them in [to jail]." As Jimena's accounts of her patients demonstrate, health-related mobility in the context of immigrant policing carries a financial premium. Ultimately mobility and cost constraints constructed through immigrant policing influenced some immigrants' decisions regarding the services they would seek.

Avoiding Services

For many undocumented immigrants in the United States, mental health services are typically inaccessible due to their high cost and the low availability of Spanish-speaking counselors (Sullivan and Rehm 2005). In Atlanta, however, there is a mental health service organization that provides services at a reduced cost to all Latinxs regardless of documentation status. Staff at this organization, Bienestar Total, noticed that after HB 87 passed some of their clients no longer sought mental health services or were forced to limit their visits. As Emma, one staff member, explained, "The main access the police got to undocumented individuals was through their car, that was the main way, . . . so many people walked, and a lot of people would spend extra money on taxi services." Spending money on taxis, as Emma explained, meant immigrants had to make strategic decisions about their finances:

> What happens when you spend money on stupid things that you really don't need to spend money on because you don't have a car? What happens is you lose money because you have to buy food, you have to put your money where it belongs, but this extra money that you could be putting towards your children's shoes or their clothes, or their education, is going to the taxi services because you are too afraid to drive. If they don't have enough money to buy shoes and necessities, do think that they are going to care about mental health services? That is just not on the top of their list; [they're thinking] "I will deal with that issue later, right now I need to deal with the food that I need to put on the table and that makes sense." And it makes sense to me, too.

For Emma, such a decision to no longer seek mental health services in an immigrant-policing context was especially disheartening because she felt these services were needed most. "At a time when everyone's so afraid, and so anxious—we get kids scared their mom and dad will get deported—that's when they need us, but they can't afford [to take a taxi] and they can't drive here."

Just as some immigrants no longer sought services at Bienestar Total, others also limited or ceased seeking services addressing intimate partner violence (IPV). One IPV service provider, Ana, recalled how women stopped coming to her support groups because the groups were held far from the women's homes. "After these laws started passing less and less women were coming to our meetings. Some of them would take the bus but it would be a whole day riding the bus for some of them and they'd get there and then they'd have to do it all over again." Eventually Ana and her organization stopped providing the IPV support groups because fewer and fewer women attended. "The sad part is that all those immigration laws and men losing their jobs meant that there was worse violence because tensions were so high," Ana added, expressing that when women needed the IPV services most, the organization could no longer offer them because women felt unsafe driving on the roads and did not want to risk deportation for seeking help with their violent home lives.

Changing Individual Health Behaviors

Not only did immigrant policing change some immigrants' mobility through vehicles, it also impacted individual health behaviors. For example, Rosa, a middle-aged woman with arthritis, engaged in low-impact exercise to stay healthy.[2] Enjoying Georgia's climate, Rosa typically exercised outside by walking through her neighborhood. "I have arthritis and I'm trying to stay healthy," Rosa explained to me when I met with her and her husband, Eduardo. "My doctor recommended I go for walks, so I try to go for walks every day." Rosa and Eduardo live in a suburban town outside of Atlanta in one of the 287(g) counties known for having an aggressive police department. Eduardo provides the primary source of income for their family since Rosa's severe arthritis limits the kind of work she can do. During one of her daily walks, a patrol car started following Rosa. "Is it a crime to walk through a neighborhood?" Rosa asked me while recalling the story of being followed. When she saw the patrol car, Rosa remembered news stories of immigrants who were arrested while walking after HB 87 passed because they could not provide a driver's licenses upon request. "I didn't know what to do—I didn't know if they could arrest me for walking or if it was a crime." Fearing the officer would stop her, Rosa walked through a side yard of a house and continued walking behind houses until she got to her own home, avoiding sidewalks and roadways where the patrol car could see her.

When she and I met, Rosa told me that walking is the only type of exercise she can do because her arthritis makes high-impact activities painful and they may harm her joints. Despite recognizing the need to exercise and knowing the only type of exercise she can engage in is walking, Rosa explained that policing might stop her from continuing her preventive health behavior. "I walk because my doctor recommended it since I'm a little overweight and have arthritis. . . . If the police start following me around all the time, I won't be able to go out anymore. How will I exercise?" Rosa's situation was further complicated following Eduardo's recent arrest for driving without a license; his immigration status was discovered, and he now faces a deportation charge. "We're here [in Atlanta] for Rosa's treatment," Eduardo explained. "Here she can get the treatment she needs." Rosa regularly receives cortisone injections to relieve the symptoms of her arthritis, but she and Eduardo claimed they would not be able to receive this type of care in the part of Mexico where they are from. If Eduardo is deported, Rosa is unsure how she will be able to afford the cortisone shots and is uncertain of what type of exercise she could perform.

Rosa's situation underscores how immigrant policing directly impacts immigrants' mobility in deeply personal ways that shape their individual health. Prior to seeing a patrol car in her neighborhood, Rosa had followed her physician's direction to engage in daily forms of exercise—but doing so exposed her to police scrutiny, which led her to stop her exercise regimen. Situations like Rosa's demonstrate how immigrant policing affects immigrants' lives, and these consequences have served as rallying cries for immigrant rights organizations.

Organizational Responses

Immigrant rights groups across Atlanta have responded to policing efforts by leading know-your-rights campaigns, organizing marches and rallies to demand political change, and engaging in public and political dialogue about immigration reform. Additionally, some service providers devised strategies for how best to reach immigrant populations while recognizing new constraints on the population's mobility due to immigrant-policing initiatives. One organization in particular, Buena Salud para Todos, offered basic sexual health programs to Latinx families and provided contraception-education services. The organization, operating out of a local multiservice center, saw a decline in program participants that one leader, Marcela, attributed to immigrant-policing initiatives. As a result, Marcela changed the organization's strategy for disseminating sexual health education and promoting contraceptive devices by offering to go to immigrants' homes. "Instead of them coming to us, we go to them!" She explained. Marcela and her staff countered concerns about driving and reduced the cost burden of attending her organization's events by leveraging the privilege of having a mobile health service program: "We go to people's houses and we tell them to call over all their neighbors and kids and we do condom demonstrations, talk about birth control, sexually transmitted diseases, and all that stuff." The necessity to "go to them," as Marcela explained, was directly related to immigrant policing altering immigrants' mobility. Accordingly, Buena Salud para Todos resisted efforts to control immigrants' lives through restricting their mobility by becoming a mobile service provider.

Just as Buena Salud para Todos adopted new mobility-related strategies to fulfill its goal, so did Bienestar Total. As part of its overall effort to promote good mental health, Bienestar Total features an after-school program for drug and alcohol prevention. The program provides a space for Latinx children to complete their homework as part of a larger goal to ensure academic success and reduce children's possible exposure to situations that could lead to drug and alcohol use. After the implementation of Georgia's harsh immigration regimes, parents of children participating in Bienestar Total's after-school program reported not wanting to have their children participate in the program because they would have to drive to pick them up and they feared possibly encountering police. In response, Bienestar Total leaders purchased buses to transport the children from school to the organization's facility and then to their parents' homes. "We got a grant to buy the buses so we can take care of transportation. . . . That means the parents don't have to worry about getting arrested [and then deported] for picking up their kids," Bienestar Total's president explained.

Organizations like Buena Salud para Todos and Bienestar Total provide examples of how specific health organizations can resist efforts to harm undocumented immigrants' overall access to social services through altering their mobility. These organizations further provide examples of mobility-specific responses to immigrant policing, but not without limitations. Not all health conditions and services can be addressed through the mobility-specific solutions employed by Buena Salud para Todos and Bienestar Total. While these programs offer alternatives to some immigrants, not all organizations have resources to support traveling staff or to purchase buses. Despite these limitations, however, these organizations' efforts suggest that harsh immigrant-policing efforts can be combated, through making certain types of services more accessible by altering the conditions in which mobility is a factor. Rather than placing burdens of mobility on clients, these organizations assume the responsibility for getting their clients to their services.

Some individual providers have, like these organizations, responded to immigrant-policing efforts in ways that make their services more accessible to undocumented patients. One provider who operates a private OB/GYN clinic, for example, has consciously kept her office near a bus route. "Some of [my patients] will come via taxi and some of them will come via bus, so I stayed here because of that," she explained. This provider serves a large number of Latinx immigrant patients, many of whom are undocumented, and thus moving to a location without bus access would limit the ability of some of her patients to see her. Organizations' and providers' responses listed here suggest how community-based responses to immigration regimes can resist efforts that restrict undocumented Latinx immigrants' mobility and impact their overall well-being.

Mobility and Forced Attrition

Immigration and mobility are connected in ways linked to rights, citizenship, and immigration into the United States. Intervening on migrants' mobility alters immigrants' resources, affects where they are able to go, and shapes an overall sense of belonging linked to place and movement (Winton 2015). Immigrant-policing regimes directly impact undocumented Latinx immigrants' sense of belonging by legislatively denying forms of movement made possible through driver's licenses and by making everyday spaces such as roadways possible sites of deportation. Law enforcement practices and programs such as Secure Communities and 287(g) impact immigrants' mobility by moving the danger of apprehension and harm concomitant with border spaces inward and into everyday space (Coleman 2012), emphasizing the mobility of the "border" as a political tool for rendering certain groups of immigrants immobile. As findings in this chapter show, immigrant policing not only raises anxieties, produces feelings of not belonging, and increases fears of deportation, but also directly impacts the health of some immigrants.

Two consequences of immigrant policing in Atlanta include changed health behaviors and use of a parallel medical system comprising informal providers and spaces seen as safe for care (Kline 2017). Since the goal of harsh immigration-enforcement regimes is to use law enforcement to encourage undocumented immigrants to "self-deport," social scientists and public health officials must do more to understand how such immigrant-policing efforts work. As the experiences of undocumented immigrants in Atlanta highlight, a key feature of immigration-enforcement regimes is the way in which they restrict mobility, broadly conceived. It is unsurprising that immigrant-policing efforts attempt to "force attrition" through restricting immigrants' mobility, since mobility is a key indicator in health-related quality of life, and punitive immigration-enforcement efforts operate to ensure that immigrants experience a poor quality of life. However, limited mobility resulting from immigrant policing sheds light on how policy can be an underlying mechanism of health inequality demanding corrective action.

Given the way in which immigrant policing directly impacts health-related mobility, social scientists and public health workers must support policy efforts that improve immigrants' mobility. Such policy efforts include granting driver's licenses to undocumented immigrants, which would allow them to traverse public roadways without risk of apprehension and deportation and would increase their ability to seek services such as IPV support and basic healthcare. Similarly, at a community level, public health agencies with grant-funding mechanisms must support actions aimed at responding to mobility-reducing immigration laws and policies. This can include offering funding for transportation services to existing organizations like Bienestar Total, which was able to continue offering services because it secured funding for transportation. These suggestions, however, are only stopgap measures, until comprehensive immigration reform passes in the United States.

Though immigration-enforcement regimes affect undocumented immigrants' mobility, they can impact their lives in such extreme ways because of undocumented immigrants' vulnerable social position based on their legal status. As undocumented immigrants have become a racialized, criminal "other" seen as undeserving of social services and forced to live their lives in fear as a result of harsh immigration regimes, sweeping immigration reform is needed to begin reversing structural vulnerabilities that directly impact the health of this population. Though comprehensive reform may not reverse all of the consequences of harsh immigrant policing, such as the trauma associated with being under a constant threat of deportation, it nevertheless may provide an opportunity to lift some of the structural, mobility-related constraints impacting undocumented immigrants' well-being.

Conclusion

While undocumented immigrants in the United States have historically experienced barriers to accessing health services and, in some situations, have avoided seeking care because they fear having their immigration status discovered (Winton 2015), immigrant policing adds another layer to existing challenges in accessing and seeking health services by leveraging roadways as places of immigration enforcement. The relationship between immigration-enforcement efforts, mobility, and the health of undocumented Latinx immigrants demands policy and research interventions. Echoing other public health scholars who have called for automobility-focused interventions, such as driver's licenses for undocumented immigrants (Rhodes et al. 2015), I assert a need for legislation that permits undocumented immigrants the ability to drive without fear of deportation. Granting safe access to navigate roadways, however, is only a small policy solution, and more sweeping immigration reforms are needed to address significant issues of fear and deportation related to immigrant policing. In addition to policy action, additional research is needed on the ways in which mobility is not only a health determinant, but also can be determined by numerous social, political, and economic factors. There is thus a need for sustained research attention to the determinants of mobility itself, and such research attention must be attentive to how mobility constraints are directly tied to health outcomes and influenced by specific political objectives like encouraging one group of people to "self-deport," which ultimately alters their health behaviors because of their efforts to avoid police.

In addition to highlighting needed interventions, findings in this chapter speak to the importance of mobile methodologies. By engaging in multisited ethnography, I aimed to understand the pathways of immigrant policing and ultimately was able to map macro-level policies to micro-level experiences through reported changes in mobility because of concerns regarding police encounters. Multisited ethnography may be one way of overcoming challenges related to connecting macro- and micro-level realities (Marcus 1995). Furthermore, findings in this chapter suggest how multisited methodology may be an important factor in activist research focused on mobility. My ability to engage in a form of "mobile ethnography" through my multisited methodology allowed me to meet undocumented immigrants in their homes and in places most comfortable to them, effectively reducing their risk of exposure to police because I met them in a space where they did not need to drive. Driving to immigrants' homes and removing one possible moment of risk for having their immigration status discovered reflects how activist scholars can leverage mobility as a tool in order to further make research processes equitable and reduce burdens imposed on vulnerable populations like undocumented immigrants.

Nolan Kline, PhD, MPH, is an assistant professor in the Department of Anthropology at Rollins College. He received a PhD in applied anthropology and an MPH from the University of South Florida. His primary research areas include immigrant policing, im/migrant health, health policy, and Latinx activism following the Pulse club shooting in Orlando, Florida. As an applied medical anthropologist, much of his work is at the interaction of health, policy, and activism, and is informed by theories of biopolitics, critical race theory, and the political economy of health.

NOTES

1. Latinx is a gender-inclusive way of referring to someone with ties to Latin America.
2. I have described Rosa's story in Kline 2017.

REFERENCES

Alcántara, Carmela, Chih-Nan Chen, and Margarita Alegría. 2014. "Do Post-migration Perceptions of Social Mobility Matter for Latino Immigrant Health?" *Social Science & Medicine* 101: 94–106.

Alexander, William L., and Magdalena Fernandez. 2014. "Immigration Policing and Medical Care for Farmworkers: Uncertainties and Anxieties in the East Coast Migrant Stream." *North American Dialogue* 17(1): 13–30.

Allen, Brian, Erica M. Cisneros, and Alexandra Tellez. 2015. "The Children Left Behind: The Impact of Parental Deportation on Mental Health." *Journal of Child and Family Studies* 24(2): 386–392.

Amuedo-Dorantes, Catalina, Thitima Puttitanun, and Ana P. Martinez-Donate. 2013. "How Do Tougher Immigration Measures Affect Unauthorized Immigrants?" *Demography* 50(3): 1067–1091.

Beckmann, Jörg. 2001. "Automobility—A Social Problem and Theoretical Concept." *Environment and Planning D: Society and Space* 19(5): 593–607.

Böhm, Steffen, Campbell Jones, Chris Land, and Mat Paterson. 2006. "Introduction: Impossibilities of Automobility." *Sociological Review* 54(Suppl. s1): 1–16.

Büscher, Monika, and John Urry. 2009. "Mobile Methods and the Empirical." *European Journal of Social Theory* 12(1): 99–116.

Cardano, Mario, Giuseppe Costa, and Moreno Demaria. 2004. "Social Mobility and Health in the Turin Longitudinal Study." *Social Science & Medicine* 58(8): 1563–1574.

Coleman, Mathew. 2012. "The 'Local' Migration State: The Site-Specific Devolution of Immigration Enforcement in the US South." *Law & Policy* 34(2): 159–190.

Cresswell, Tim. 2006. *On the Move: Mobility in the Modern Western World.* London: Routledge.

———. 2010. "Towards a Politics of Mobility." *Environment and Planning D: Society and Space* 28(1): 17–31.

Dahl, Espen. 1996. "Social Mobility and Health: Cause or Effect?" *BMJ: British Medical Journal* 313(7055): 435–436.

Dreby, Joanna. 2012. "The Burden of Deportation on Children in Mexican Immigrant Families." *Journal of Marriage and Family* 74(4): 829–845.

Foucault, Michel. 2003. *Society Must Be Defended: Lectures at the Collége de France, 1975–76.* New York: Picador.

Gwyther, Marni E., and Melinda Jenkins. 1998. "Migrant Farmworker Children: Health Status, Barriers to Care, and Nursing Innovations in Health Care Delivery." *Journal of Pediatric Health Care* 12(2): 60–66.

Hacker, Karen, Jocelyn Chu, Carolyn Leung, Robert Marra, Alex Pirie, Mohamed Brahimi, Margaret English, Joshua Beckmann, Dolores Acevedo-Garcia, and Robert P.

Marlin. 2011. "The Impact of Immigration and Customs Enforcement on Immigrant Health: Perceptions of Immigrants in Everett, Massachusetts, USA." *Social Science & Medicine* 73(4): 586–594.

Hale, C. R. 2006. "Activist Research v. Cultural Critique: Indigenous Land Rights and the Contradictions of Politically Engaged Anthropology." *Cultural Anthropology* 21(1): 96–120.

Hardy, Lisa J., Christina M. Getrich, Julio C. Quezada, Amanda Guay, Raymond J. Michalowski, and Eric Henley. 2012. "A Call for Further Research on the Impact of State-Level Immigration Policies on Public Health." *American Journal of Public Health* 102(7): 1250–1253.

Kline, Nolan. 2017. "Pathogenic Policy: Immigrant Policing, Fear, and Parallel Medical Systems in the US South." *Medical Anthropology* 36(4): 396–410.

Kobach, Kris W. 2008. "Attrition through Enforcement: A Rational Approach to Illegal Immigration." *Tulane Journal of International and Comparative Law* 15: 155–163.

Mao, Liang, Jeanne-Marie R. Stacciarini, Rebekah Smith, and Brenda Wiens. 2015. "An Individual-Based Rurality Measure and Its Health Application: A Case Study of Latino Immigrants in North Florida, USA." *Social Science & Medicine* 147: 300–308.

Marcus, George E. 1995. "Ethnography in/of the World System: The Emergence of Multi-Sited Ethnography." *Annual Review of Anthropology* 24: 95–117.

Menjívar, Cecilia. 2014. "The 'Poli-Migra': Multilayered Legislation, Enforcement Practices, and What We Can Learn About and From Today's Approaches." *American Behavioral Scientist* 58(13): 1–15.

Pulido, Laura. 2008. "FAQs: Frequently (Un)asked Questions about Being a Scholar Activist." In *Engaging Contradictions: Theory, Politics, and Methods of Activist Scholarship*, ed. Charles R. Hale, 341–365. Berkeley, CA: University of California Press.

Quesada, James, Laurie Kain Hart, and Philippe Bourgois. 2011. "Structural Vulnerability and Health: Latino Migrant Laborers in the United States." *Medical Anthropology* 30(4): 339–362.

Rhodes, Scott D., Lilli Mann, Florence M. Simán, Eunyoung Song, Jorge Alonzo, Mario Downs, Emma Lawlor, Omar Martinez, Christina J. Sun, and Mary Claire O'Brien. 2015. "The Impact of Local Immigration Enforcement Policies on the Health of Immigrant Hispanics/Latinos in the United States." *American Journal of Public Health* 105(2): 329–337.

Sheller, Mimi. 2004. "Automotive Emotions: Feeling the Car." *Theory, Culture & Society* 21(4/5): 221–242.

Sheller, Mimi, and John Urry. 2000. "The City and the Car." *International Journal of Urban and Regional Research* 24(4): 737–757.

Stuesse, Angela, and Mathew Coleman. 2014. "Automobility, Immobility, Altermobility: Surviving and Resisting the Intensification of Immigrant Policing." *City & Society* 26(1): 105–126.

Su, Rick. 2012. "The States of Immigration." *William & Mary Law Review* 54(4): 1339–1407.

Sullivan, M. M., and R. Rehm. 2005. "Mental Health of Undocumented Mexican Immigrants: A Review of the Literature." *Advances in Nursing Science* 28(3): 240.

Weathers, Andrea, Cynthia Minkovitz, Patricia O'Campo, and Marie Diener-West. 2003. "Health Services Use by Children of Migratory Agricultural Workers: Exploring the Role of Need for Care." *Pediatrics* 111(5): 956–963.

White, Kari, Valerie A. Yeager, Nir Menachemi, and Isabel C. Scarinci. 2014. "Impact of Alabama's Immigration Law on Access to Health Care among Latina Immigrants and Children: Implications for National Reform." *American Journal of Public Health* 104(3): 397–405.

Wilson, Astrid Hellier, Judith Lupo Wold, Lorine Spencer, and Kathleen Pittman. 2000. "Primary Health Care for Hispanic Children of Migrant Farm Workers." *Journal of Pediatric Health Care* 14(5): 209–215.

Winton, Ailsa. 2015. "Violence, Borders, and Boundaries: Reframing Young People's Mobility." In *Movement, Mobilities, and Journeys: Geographies of Children and Young People*, ed. Caitriona Ni Laoire, Allen White, and Tracey Skelton, 1–19. Singapore: Springer.

Wullems, Jorgen A., Sabine M.P. Verschueren, Hans Degens, Christopher I. Morse, and Gladys L. Onambélé. 2016. "A Review of the Assessment and Prevalence of Sedentarism in Older Adults, Its Physiology/Health Impact and Non-exercise Mobility Counter-Measures." *Biogerontology* 17(3): 1–19.

Zapata Roblyer, Martha I., Joseph G. Grzywacz, Cynthia K. Suerken, Grisel Trejo, Edward H. Ip, Thomas A. Arcury, and Sara A. Quandt. 2015. "Interpersonal and Social Correlates of Depressive Symptoms among Latinas in Farmworker Families Living in North Carolina." *Women & Health* 56(2): 1–17.

CHAPTER 3

(Im)mobile Populations and Health Rights

Accessing the Healthcare System in Slovenia

Uršula Lipovec Čebron and Sara Pistotnik

In the fall of 2015 and winter of 2016, a few hundred thousand refugees crossed Slovenia via the so-called Balkan route.[1] Despite knowing in advance that the refugees taking the Balkan route would travel through Slovenia if the Hungarian state closed its borders, Slovene government institutions remained unprepared. Immediately after the refugees' arrival, many people from Slovenia mobilized and helped as volunteers in crucial areas. The Slovene government, on the other hand, established a discourse of securitization (Huysmans 2000) in the language of a "refugee crisis," which presented refugees as a security threat to Slovene residents. As a result, something that would probably never have been accepted by Slovene residents a couple of years earlier became normalized: the army was given additional powers over border control, a barbed wire fence was established on the southern border with the Republic of Croatia, and more than 400,000 refugees were held at reception centers.[2] In these centers, they often suffered intolerable and unhygienic living conditions (sleeping outdoors in the cold during the winter, being held for many hours without food and water, having access to few or no toilets, being enclosed and assaulted by police, etc.). As a result, the refugees were constantly exposed to life-threatening situations and severe health risks (Mirovni inštitut 2015).

Under such conditions, the quality of healthcare was also inadequate. A medical worker helping refugees established that

> the quality of medical care was insufficient. . . . Due to the lack of adequate medical facilities, some experienced treating patients in such terrible conditions, such as on the hard ground and in the mud. . . . Many of them faced lack of human resources, as well as medical material and technical capacity to cope with the large number of patients. . . . Lack of resources and high fluctuation of patients resulted in rapid assessments and medication prescriptions. (Jazbinšek et al. 2016)

Even though this situation was in many respects specific, the insufficient access to quality healthcare for migrants and refugees in Slovenia is not an exception to the rule. Claims of inadequate and poorly accessible healthcare for refugees date back two decades and are supported by statements of asylum seekers, undocumented migrants, and other migrants that live in Slovenia, as well as the residents who were erased from the permanent residence registry. In addition, their experiences are confirmed by a recently published analysis of migrants' access to healthcare, which ranked Slovenia at the penultimate place among thirty-eight countries:

> SI [Slovenia] does almost nothing to integrate and orient newcomer patients into the health system and to address any of their specific health needs. Its targeted health policies are . . . far below average even for Central Europe. Health services are only made accessible and responsive to newcomer patients by providing information on their legal entitlements and, if they are lucky, an interpreter. Even these rather favorable legal entitlements can be blocked in practice by providers making discretionary decisions and requests for documentation. (MIPEX 2015)

How is this possible in a country that provided de facto universal access to healthcare for all its residents prior to 1991? What is the basis for the paradigmatic shift of the welfare state, from a society where improving health was one of the main goals to a society where healthcare is seen as an individual's responsibility? How should we understand a breach between the declarative position of governmental institutions claiming health insurance is still accessible to all residents and an increasing number of individuals without health insurance, among them many migrants and refugees? In this chapter we point out some of the factors that have led to the present situation, in which Slovenia has introduced increasingly unequal and unhealthy health policies (Castro and Singer 2004). This includes the important role that regulated mobility of a number of Slovene residents played in legitimation of more restricted access to public institutions including the healthcare system.

From Universality to Selectivity

Before we analyze the increasingly restrictive access to the Slovene healthcare system, we have to consider larger societal processes occurring in this region in the last twenty-five years. These processes, which have greatly influenced cutbacks in healthcare rights, emerged shortly after Slovene independence. They represent a paradigmatic change in the welfare state and the implementation of new management of mobility in the framework of European migration policies.

In Slovenia before 1991, a socialist model of the welfare state was implemented that differed significantly from its Western counterpart. In contrast to its liberal alternative in Western societies, the Yugoslav socialist welfare state, in many respects, aimed to intervene in the very sources of social inequality, and for this particular purpose, it employed policies based on the notion of universality. The socialist state regulation thus established social consensus through the combination of permanent employment of the active population, opportunities for social mobility, and universal access to social rights.

After Slovenian independence in 1991, a change in the social system took place, influenced by structural adjustments related to the goal of joining the European integration. Part of this process has been a slow disintegration of the former state regulation, moving away from the notion of universality, but this trend is characteristic not only of Slovenia. Over the course of several decades, we have witnessed a restructuring of the Western capitalist system that has been restoring the means of production and exploitation of wealth, and subsequently the relations of power, to a pre–World War II situation (Burcar 2012: 225). These processes aim to restore the absolute power and wealth of the capitalist elites that, in the 1970s, found new means of acquiring profit due to the stagnation of traditional modes of production and exhausted possibilities for the expansion of profits (Burcar 2012; MSU and Akademska solidarnost 2012). One strategic move was an organized attack on labor rights and on the mechanisms of the welfare state. The latter became a target of many critics—starting with the neoclassical economic perspective, which advocates that "the 'generous' state discourages people from work, decreases the employment rate and increases expenses for social transfers, which leads to lower growth rate, lower wages and consequently to increased levels of poverty" (Leskošek 2013, 149). The negative effects of the welfare state, leading to a lower growth rate, are, indeed, highly disputable, and the empirical evidence suggests a positive linkage between welfare states and lower risks of poverty. Nevertheless, the neoclassical economic arguments seem to prevail, questioning the fair redistribution of goods and social rights, posing a danger to social consensus. The arguments also advocate a paradigmatic shift (Leskošek 2013: 149) that foretells the end of the welfare state as we know it.

Inda (2006) claims that the concept of the welfare state in Western societies was gradually replaced with that of a post-social state, where the government is no longer required to plan, know, and direct from the center to address a society's desire for health, security, and other issues that were previously addressed by the mechanisms of the welfare state. "The responsibility for dealing with these problems is therefore largely displaced from the state to the multitude of specific actors: individuals, schools, communities, localities, hospitals, charities, and so forth" (Inda 2006: 12–13). If the individual's rights and obligations emerged from collective solidarity and social responsibility (which was the case in the welfare state), where the individual and the state were bound to a reciprocal mechanism of rights and duties, the post-social regimes of government differed in the sense that one's security did not emerge primarily from collective rights, but rather from an active care for one's own life, enterprise, and self-promotion (Inda 2006: 15). Other authors have also addressed the problem of transferring the state's responsibility onto the individual (Leskošek 2013; Leskošek et al. 2013; Peck 2001). Instead of addressing one's rights, dignity, and needs, the discourse now focuses on individual responsibility, self-sufficiency, and empowerment (Leskošek 2013: 164).

Within a post-social context, the increasing loss of social rights is often legitimized by discrediting anyone who differs from the ideal of the post-social resident. Discourses in the field of social policies clearly show the construction of the Other through discrimination, disqualification, and criminalization of individuals who are either asserting their social rights or unable to exercise them despite their aggravated social position. This is taking place by employing a historical dichotomy of "deserving" and "undeserving" residents, the former being described as responsible or "ethical," diligent, and hard-working taxpayers, while the latter are commonly denoted as irresponsible or "unethical," thieves, idlers, and exploiters (see Horton 2004; Inda 2006: 46–47; Leskošek et al. 2013: 204).

In addition, it is important to point out that social rights are historically linked to the development of nation-states. Social rights advanced greatly after World War II, when the uncontested division of territory among nation-states most notably constituted the core of the world order at that time (Bauman 2005). As a result, membership in a certain community is nowadays attested by citizenship status or by permanent residence, upon which one's social rights and contributions depend (Leskošek 2016: 93). In order to assert one's social rights, identification as a member of the community is crucial, while a line is established between citizens and foreigners.

After Slovene independence this line became a very sensitive issue. With the formation and later collapse of the former Yugoslavia, "borders and relations between people and places changed, and these changes have had grave effects on the (im)mobility of people" (Gregorič Bon and Repič 2016: 1). In the 1990s, Slovenia introduced new migration management that was driven by structural adjustments in order to become part of the European Union. One of the important motivations behind these changes was a promise of free mobility. In reality, this process was not so straightforward. Emanating from a simple distinction between citizens and foreigners, European policies suddenly enabled a wide spectrum of status options (e.g., undocumented person, individual with provisional retention permit, asylum seeker, person granted subsidiary protection, refugee, individual with a temporary residence permit, person with a permanent residence permit, citizen). The scope of rights and duties of individuals within this hierarchy was determined, to a larger or smaller degree, by the closeness of the relationship between an individual and the state. The greatest number of rights was accorded to citizens, and the smallest number of rights—or rather no rights at all—to undocumented migrants (Pistotnik 2010: 57).

Lack of rights has a huge influence on a person's mobility. As other authors have shown (Cresswell 2006, 2010; see also Castañeda's and Kline's chapters in this book), undocumented migrants and other migrants with precarious status face restrictions in mobility (being unable to move freely in a territory or cross its borders) as well as experience different forms of exclusion, which results in socially immobile individuals. Thus, the effect of European migration policies was that "European citizens became mobile, and as a consequence non-European citizens became immobile (blocked, stopped, prevented)" (Tuccillo Castaldo 2007: 141; see also Cresswell 2006; Sheller and Urry 2006; Khan 2016). A sharp distinction was introduced among Slovene residents, generating persons with different kinds of mobility—either encouraged or restricted. Even more, due to a lesser scope of rights, restricted mobility was accelerated and reproduced by more limited access to public institutions, which were being transformed from universality to selectivity.

In this chapter, we demonstrate how social rights in the post-social state are being diminished: first, those rights affecting noncitizens (i.e., migrants) and, later on, those affecting economically underprivileged residents (e.g., precarious workers, unemployed people, the poor). In addition, we will show how the process of exclusion is closely linked to the production of the

Other as an undeserving individual, one who is—in accordance with the neoliberal logic of selection—facing a rapid reduction in his or her rights. This will be analyzed within the context of increasingly restrictive access to health insurance and urgent treatment in Slovenia, where the largest population of migrants who suddenly lost their rights in the 1990s were former permanent residents, whose status changed even though they did not migrate anywhere. The article is based on ethnographic research that took place from 2005 to 2016.[3] The research focused generally on the transformation of the welfare state in independent Slovenia and on different health-related issues experienced by (im)mobilized populations (e.g., migrants/refugees, erased persons, precarious workers), especially their access to Slovenia's healthcare system.

Reforming the Healthcare System

> Before the adoption of a capitalist orientation in the Slovene healthcare system we regularly did medical checkups for people without health insurance, as for everybody else. Even the doctors' referrals for further procedures were never denied, unlike today when they are denied with the argument that there is no coverage by health insurance. However, in the beginning of 1990s, with the new labor conditions and this new capitalist orientation, the difficulties began for all patients with no health insurance
>
> —Dr Aleksander Doplihar, GP

As is clear from the quotation above, the healthcare system of former Yugoslavia was generally accessible to all residents, including individuals who did not have health insurance or did not pay health contributions (Lipovec Čebron 2011a, 2011b; Markota et al. 1999; Toth 2003). Consequently, the whole population of the former Yugoslavia was entitled to almost any kind of medical assistance, mostly without additional fees (Markota et al. 1999: 2). After Slovene independence, a different perspective prevailed, which emphasized that universal accessibility to the healthcare system was financially untenable due to almost unlimited healthcare rights and the impossibility of covering the costs of an increasingly expensive healthcare system (Markota and Albreht 2001: 20). Although these arguments do not seem very convincing in the context of current indebtedness (see, e.g., Majcen and Čok 2014: 62), they contributed significantly to a radical change in the Slovene healthcare system. One of the crucial aspects of this change was conditional access to the healthcare system within a new health insurance scheme, which established two types of insurance: first, compulsory health insurance, which is obligatory for Slovene citizens with permanent residence in Slovenia, but does not cover all costs of treatment (full coverage of costs is ensured only for children, for students up to age twenty-six who regularly attend school, and in the case of certain diagnoses and conditions); and second, complementary health insurance, which is voluntary and covers the difference between the full price of health services and the percentage covered by compulsory health insurance.[4] The insurance premium for complementary health insurance is to be paid by an individual. A person who lacks complementary health insurance must pay an additional sum out of pocket for the majority of medical services. To acquire complementary health insurance, the person has to first have compulsory health insurance. This presents a serious problem for migrants and other residents, who do not have access to compulsory health insurance.

The new health insurance scheme was also the basis for reformed financing of the healthcare system. Specifically, compulsory health insurance provides the largest source of the healthcare budget, and the majority of this share is based on contributions from workers' salaries (and other personal incomes) and from employers (Kersnik 2001). Thus, most Slovene citizens and migrants acquire their health insurance on the basis of employment, whereas local communities provide financial resources for socially disadvantaged individuals (citizens and migrants with permanent residence permits).

In addition to linking the healthcare budget directly with employment, the healthcare reform opened a new chapter for the privatization of healthcare and the emergence of additional payments for various medical services, remedies, equipment, and medication. The present system offers certain benefits, such as a promise of full coverage for the population with compulsory health insurance (at least on a declarative level) and continuity of contributions that are defined progressively according to personal income. Nonetheless, the reformed healthcare system enabled further inequality with regards to accessibility to healthcare services. Services of the welfare state that were once universal now pose a new source of inequality and exclusion (Zorn 2010: 39). Even the Slovene Constitution does not protect against the shift from universal healthcare access to selective access. Specifically, Article 51 (Right to Health Care) states no assurance of one's universal health rights, nor of a right to free medical treatment. "According to the Slovenian Constitution, all rights in relation to one's health are put into effect by law, which can put new conditions on the claims to, and realization of, these rights. However, the obligation of the state to assure health insurance is limited to citizens only. As a result, the state directly interferes with the universality of rights that are derived from the very purpose of health insurance" (Rajgelj 2012: 44).

Public institutions seemingly unconnected with migration management reproduce its logic of exclusion and contribute to mechanisms of immobilization of migrants. The public healthcare system does not admit *everyone,* only *some* groups of people. Initial selection runs on the basis of access to health insurance: *some* people have access to compulsory, as well as complementary, health insurance, while others do not. The criteria for this selection, which consequently lead to exclusion of some, are (1) citizenship or permanent residence in the Republic of Slovenia, or (2) regular employment (permanent or part-time).

Excluding Noncitizens from the Health Insurance System

> I paid for everything, but they still asked me all sorts of things, how come I don't have a medical card, but they didn't believe me, they mused over it, and they scolded me. . . . Yes, that's what they did. "Why don't you have a medical card? Why haven't you fixed this problem?" Then, when I explained to them, they didn't believe me and still said, "Well, why haven't you fixed it?"
>
> —Jana S., erased person

As already stated, access to health rights became limited to those with citizenship status in the early 1990s. The most obvious example of this radical change was "the erased": the first (and most populous) group of individuals without health insurance in newly independent Slovenia. The erased are people who were born in Slovenia or had migrated there from one of the former Yugoslav republics. Many came to Slovenia in the 1960s and 1970s as internal migrants (from other republics of the former federation) in response to a growing demand for workers in Slovenian companies. All of them had permanent residence status in Slovenia and enjoyed access to the rights of all citizens, including health rights.

After Slovenia's declaration of independence in 1991, the newly formed Slovenian authorities set up a new nation-state apparatus, starting with the redefinition of its citizens. Since they decided to apply a principle of continuity with past republican citizenship, the majority of the population—who held citizenship of the former Yugoslav Socialist Republic of Slovenia—automatically were granted citizenship of the newly established country (Dedič, Jalušič, and Zorn 2003; Zorn and Lipovec Čebron 2007).

However, for those who were citizens of any other former Yugoslav republic, a period of six months was set for the submission of citizenship applications. The status of individuals who failed to do so, or whose applications were rejected, changed abruptly. On 26 February 1992, the Slovenian Ministry of Interior Affairs erased them from the Registry of Permanent Residents of the Republic of Slovenia and annulled all the rights that these permanent residents had once possessed—making them essentially equivalent to undocumented migrants. As a result, 25,671 individuals (more than 1 percent of Slovenia's population) lost all social, economic, and political rights (Dedič et al. 2003; Kogovšek and Petkovič 2010) without changing their place of residence; that is, they became regarded as migrants without migrating anywhere. Immobility, or "stuckness, being in-between" (Khan 2016: 98), became a permanent feature of their everyday life.

The experience described above by an erased person implies that one consequence of the erasure was also limited or denied access to healthcare services due to the absence of health insurance, because their legal status was made the equivalent of that of undocumented migrants.[5] Their experience set a precedent for a future trend of narrowing access to healthcare for many categories of migrants. As a result of Slovenia's adoption of hierarchical migration management strategies, mentioned above, all individuals who have migrated to Slovenia since the 1990s have been selectively admitted into the healthcare system. Some of them (employed migrants with permanent or temporary residence permits)[6] have legal rights to compulsory health insurance, while others (undocumented migrants, asylum seekers, individuals with provisional retention permits, unemployed persons with temporary residence permits) have no such rights.

Despite the fact that in various countries (e.g., Italy, France, the Netherlands, Switzerland, Sweden), or their respective regions, some migrant/refugee groups—undocumented migrants, asylum seekers, unemployed migrants with temporary statuses—have the right to health insurance (MIPEX 2015), access to health insurance for migrants in Slovenia is more or less conditional upon formal employment. Therefore, if the right to healthcare is inherently bestowed to residents of some EU countries based on the fact that they live in the territory of the respective state (regardless of their participation in its labor market), the Slovene selective logic legitimizes its restrictions to social rights imposed by the management of mobility by dividing people into two categories: those who "deserve" to have such right and those who are "undeserving" and thus denied this right (Becker 2004: 260; Horton 2004, 478; Leskošek 2013).

Employed migrants in Slovenia are "permitted" access to health insurance. They are perceived as "ethical" subjects (Inda 2006), as their ability to obtain employment is seen as proof of their responsibility, activity, and diligence (Becker 2004: 260; Horton 2004: 478). This enables them to pay the cost of the insurance through taxes. In contrast, unemployed migrants are considered "undeserving" of the right to health insurance, as they appear to be "unethical" subjects (Inda 2006) who are inactive and irresponsible, posing a threat of various health risks (Becker 2004: 260; Horton 2004: 478). As Kline (in this volume) shows, social and political mobilities are often questioned because of a person's migration status and articulated "undeservingness" of publicly funded health services. This dichotomy between "deserving" and "undeserving" individuals is often reinforced and justified through the notion of a "burden" that these irresponsible and unproductive individuals put on the healthcare budget. Migrants can thus exist only as a productive precarious workforce that contributes to economic growth and competitiveness (Walters 2004: 238–39); that is, "they should not pose a burden to the state with social costs, but rather contribute to the community with their work" (Verlič-Christensen 2002: 44). Similarly, Fassin (2004: 205) argues, "Most often, it is their economic function that justifies their presence, primarily through their contribution to the production of wealth as an undemanding and unorganized labor force." In reality, this corresponds to the very practical fact that the more migrants are illegalized, and thus faced with limited access to autonomous mobility and rights, the more likely they are to be exposed to exploitation and the less cost they represent for employers or the state. In cases of work loss or illness, some groups of migrants can easily be removed from the state without any possibility of re-entering it and exercising their social rights.

Even though in Slovenia this segregational logic pertaining to migrants came first, the past few years have shown that once the principle of universality was undermined, the very same notion served as an excuse for unequal access to healthcare services for an increasing number of citizens. An immediate consequence of the economic crisis and climbing rate of unemployment was an increasing competitiveness on the level of the distribution of social goods, including social housing, unemployment benefits, and other types of financial aid, together with access to healthcare (see Huysmans 2000, 2006). Therefore, from 2008 onwards, advocates of a neoclassical economic perspective used austerity measures to further disintegrate the welfare state amid its transformation into a post-social state (Inda 2006). The reduction and deficit of social rights led to further segregation in Slovenia, not only in terms of a dichotomy of citizens versus noncitizens, but also in terms of dichotomies of "productive"/"deserving" versus "unproductive"/"undeserving" individuals in general.

In a dichotomic logic driven by selection and exclusion, various legal, administrative, and practical mechanisms were established to prevent an increasing number of residents to exercise their right to health (Leskošek 2016: 96–97; Pistotnik and Lipovec Čebron 2015). In addition to migrants without a permanent residence permit, these groups comprised mainly self-employed persons, their family members, single persons, registered or unregistered same-sex partners, and the children in their families—in other words, those who diverged from existing norms in the fields of employment, family, and immigration in that they were not employed, married, or Slovene citizens (Rajgelj 2012: 51; see Pistotnik and Lipovec Čebron 2015). Therefore, the most distinctive feature of the period since 2008 is an increasing number of once "deserving" citizens who have now slipped to the bottom of the healthcare hierarchy, among the "undeserving" individuals (Huysmans 2000: 768).

In this diminishing of the right to healthcare we can see how the hierarchization of Slovene residents based on restriction of mobility and/or access to rights led to the legitimization of exclusion for non-Slovene citizens. Even more, once denied access to the healthcare system for certain groups of migrants was fully normalized in society, the same logic started to be applied not only to other residents, but also to certain medical treatments that had previously been regarded as unquestionable. In the following section, we present a case study of the state encroaching on the most basic healthcare right, the right to urgent treatment, which is still protected by law but—due to a series of sophisticated mechanisms—has become harder to assert.

Restriction of the Right to Urgent Treatment

> When accessing health services, one could argue that foreign women with provisional retention permits, with temporary residence permits, as well as women without regulated legal status represent the most vulnerable social group. Namely, the healthcare rights of all these women are limited to a single right, provisioned by law: the right to urgent treatment. We have experienced a situation when a foreign woman with a two-year temporary residence permit, yet without any income, got very sick, which led to a terminal illness (metastasized cancer). Cancer treatment is normally considered urgent treatment, but the patient faced many problems that emerged from the fact she did not have health insurance coverage at the time [of medical treatment].
>
> —Employee at a domestic violence shelter

For all uninsured persons in need of medical assistance in the Slovene territory, a "safety switch" exists that enables minimal medical assistance. For the above-mentioned groups of migrants, including the erased, and all other individuals who are unable to gain access to health insurance, there is a declaratory possibility of accessing urgent medical help and necessary treatment. Urgent treatment assumes a very limited scope of healthcare treatments, including only immediate service (emergency live-saving measures), life-sustaining treatment, and prophylaxis (measures designed to preserve health and prevent the spread of disease).[7] Even though this care is regarded as a basic, fundamental right, it is disputable whether we could even consider it a concrete right in view of its minimal scope.

More important is the question of accessibility to this right. According to the Slovenian health legislation, urgent treatment should be free of charge and universally accessible to all people, regardless of their health insurance status.[8] Yet, the above quotation and data from various studies (Lipovec Čebron 2010, 2011a, 2011b; Lipovec Čebron, Svetel and Pistotnik 2015; MIPEX 2015; Pistotnik and Lipovec Čebron 2015) reveal that the principle of selectivity seems to undermine universality, as is evident by a series of obstacles restricting access to it.

First, although the definition of urgent treatment seems to be clear and unambiguous, in practice it depends largely on an arbitrary assessment by health workers. As a result, urgent medical assistance varies greatly among different healthcare institutions across Slovenia (ranging from very restrictive to very liberal readings), leading to a potential violation of this right. The experiences of the erased people and other marginalized individuals confirm that the same medical problem may be addressed free of charge in one institution but is not addressed without fees in another (Lipovec Čebron 2011a). Since the concept of urgent medical assistance is characterized by confusion, ambiguity, and arbitrary conduct, it is not a surprising fact that the legal logic gives in to the principle of arbitrariness, mainly due to vague legal provisions (Ticktin 2006, 37). Thus, collective decisions become a matter of individual judgment.

Secondly, ethnographic research (Lipovec Čebron, Svetel, and Pistotnik 2015) shows a tendency among healthcare institutions to try to charge for urgent treatment, even when such treatment should be free of charge. This has become a practice predominantly in cases of migrants without health insurance and other persons who are unable to defend their rights and interests because of linguistic, social, economic, and other impediments.

Thirdly, the right to urgent treatment has been further limited by changes to admission guidelines for healthcare institutions from 2010 onward (Slovenia, Ministry of Health 2010a). This is reflected in the introduction of the rather complicated administrative procedure of issuing a reimbursement claim for costs of urgent treatment from the Ministry of Health. The issuing of this document requires extensive administrative work and acquisition of various pieces of evidence by health workers. As a result, the criteria to successfully conclude this procedure are often almost impossible to meet.

Finally, the right to urgent treatment was further restricted by a provision that implies personal responsibility of the primary acting doctor, who is required to sign a statement that the treatment was actually necessary and that the performer of medical assistance would, in case this were not true, reimburse any unjustified costs of the service (Slovenia, Ministry of Health 2010b). Should the treatment of an uninsured person prove to be unnecessary, and the treated person does not have sufficient funds to cover the expense of the treatment, the financial burden of the treatment becomes a liability for the healthcare professionals who administered the service (Pistotnik and Lipovec Čebron 2015).

All of these factors represent a complex web of restrictions that influence the decisions of health workers regarding urgent medical treatment, in spite of the declarative inclusiveness of health legislation, and pose a substantial threat to acknowledging this fundamental right to necessary medical assistance. Not only does urgent medical treatment represent a very limited scope of medical services, but its current arrangement creates a problem of accessibility for people without health insurance—especially in times of radical financial cutbacks and severe austerity policies and when the selective logic of who deserves access to healthcare free of charge is fully normalized in Slovene society. The practice shows that even the "safety switch," which under Slovenian law should grant access to a minimum amount of medical treatment for all, is not serving its purpose because it is not considered universal and unquestionable.

Conclusion

In this chapter, we strived to present mobility as a human activity upon which states impose various restrictions and, in doing so, regulate access to rights, including healthcare. We followed developments in Slovenia after its independence in 1991, where more restrictive regulation of mobility for non-EU citizens was one of the processes that contributed to a gradual substitution of the welfare state with a post-social state. More precisely, it helped to transform the Slovene healthcare system from universal to more selective, starting with barriers to health insurance for erased persons and migrants. This process of separation between citizens and foreigners was justified through conceptions of "deserving" and "undeserving" individuals, a logic that not only expanded further to encompass other Slovene residents, but also enhanced restrictions on once unquestionable medical treatments such as urgent medical care.

From an anthropological perspective, inequalities can be understood in terms of how societies treat their most vulnerable members. One can grasp, as its extremes, the nature of the social contract that binds human beings in a given space and defines their sense of politics (Arendt 1995 in Fassin 2004). Migrants (or foreigners) thus seem to be the "paradigmatic group of greatest liminality since they belong neither to the community of origin nor to that of the nation" (Fassin 2004: 204).

Fassin's statement can also be applied to the situation of migrants in Slovenia. As we aimed to show in the case of access to healthcare services and health insurance, the welfare state is undergoing a gradual process of disintegration. This process is most evident in the encroachment of rights of the most liminal or marginalized population groups: the erased and migrants without citizenship and/or permanent residence. The process of encroachment then advances, as a centripetal force, to other marginalized groups, in order to diminish their scope of rights as well. This, among other processes, is established through the mechanisms that produce the Other, which justify the selection of access to these rights by discriminating all socially excluded and disadvantaged people, denoting them as "undeserving" (lazy, cheating, exploiting) individuals.

Overall, the production of the Other is a complex process that occurs on many simultaneous levels and through the interaction of many agents, including public institutions. Its aim is to push various social groups to the margins in order that they become socially invisible and ever more immobilized. When public institutions fail to acknowledge these groups, they cease to feel responsible for their welfare, thus reproducing the logic of the post-social state—leaving them to be resourceful and to search for alternative options. In case they fail, the institutions usually pass on their part of responsibility to the "underprivileged" Other, blaming them for their own life decisions.

The rest of the population is unable to identify with the excluded groups, as they represent the Other; therefore, the majority of the population remain idle and unresponsive when it comes to limitations and/or encroachment of their rights. As Feldman (1996) argues, this can be an example of "cultural anesthesia," which helps to quiet down the unpleasant and contradictory circumstances, experiences, and feelings of all those individuals who are being constructed as the cultural Other. Those experiences and feelings are being silenced because should they become public and visible to others, they would threaten to undermine the normalizing and often silent premises of everyday life, as well as the legitimacy of power (Feldman 1996; see also Dedič et al. 2003). As long as residents are in the grip of "cultural anesthesia," they fail to see that the encroachment of rights belonging to a certain group of people is a definite sign of disintegration of the social system on the whole. Moreover, their idle position as passive observers enables the undisturbed continuation of encroachment of an ever-growing scope of rights and eventual consolidation of the post-social state.

Uršula Lipovec Čebron, PhD, is assistant professor in the Department of Ethnology and Cultural Anthropology, Faculty of Arts, University of Ljubljana, where she teaches several courses (e.g., Anthropology of Migration, Contemporary Migration, Ethnic Minorities and Citizenship, Medical Anthropology) and is engaged in national and international projects. In her recent scientific articles she deals with the health aspects of migration as well as erasure of residents of Slovenia; she is coeditor of several publications—including *Balkan Migration Route* (*Journal for the Critique of Science,* 2016), *Stories of Erased Citizens* (Sanje Publishing, 2011), and *Once upon an Erasure* (*Journal for the Critique of Science,* 2007)—and author of a medical anthropological book, *Crossroads of Health and Illness: Traditional and Complementary Medicines in Istria* (Ljubljana University Press, Faculty of Arts, 2008).

Sara Pistotnik, is a researcher in the Department of Ethnology and Cultural Anthropology, Faculty of Arts, University of Ljubljana. She collaborates on a number of national and international projects focused mostly on the field of migration, apatridity, erasure of residents of Slovenia, and related health aspects. Her current research interest is understanding patterns of different state mechanisms of exclusion, especially in relation to the Slovene healthcare system. She has published several scientific articles and book chapters.

NOTES

1. According to official statistics, 477,724 refugees entered the country in the period from 16 October 2015 to 11 March 2016, most of them transiting to Austria, Germany, and other European countries. The majority were fleeing from the conflicts in Syria, Afganistan, Iraq, and Iran, among others (Slovenia, Ministry of the Interior 2015).
2. Arrival camps were located along Slovene border in (among other places) Brežice, Dobova, Šentij, Gornja Radgona, Središče ob Dravi, and Petišovci.
3. For example, Uršula Lipovec Čebron's and Sara Pistotnik's research conducted in the framework of the project Together for Health (Skupaj za zdravje), National Institute for Public Health (2014–16), and research conducted in the framework of projects The Erased People of Slovenia - A Challenge of a Young Nation-State (2007–2009) and The Erased: Remedying Human Rights Violations (2010–12), Peace Institute Slovenia; Uršula Lipovec Čebron's PhD research, "Erased Residents without Medical Citizenship: A Medical Anthropological Research" (2005–11); and Sara Pistotnik's PhD research, "People without a State: Cases from the Area of Former Yugoslavia" (2013–).
4. The compulsory health insurance is provided by the Health Insurance Institute of Slovenia, which is a public institution. The complementary insurance can be arranged at one of three insurance companies. In cases of restoration of legal status

on the basis of employment, erased persons regained access to the healthcare system via health insurance through their work.

5. In addition, persons with refugee status have the right to access compulsory health insurance; since 2014, the same right is granted to individuals with permanent residence permits who meet the criteria for financial aid for the socially underprivileged.
6. Urgent treatment comprises immediate treatment after emergency medical assistance, nursing (wound dressing), prevention of sudden and fatal deteriorations of chronic diseases or health conditions that could lead to severe damage of respective organs and/or their functions, etc. (Article No. 103, Compulsory Health Insurance Regulation (Pravila obveznega zdravstvenega zavarovanja)).
7. As per the Health Care and Health Insurance Act (Zakon o zdravstvenem varstvu in zdravstvenem zavarovanju), everyone, regardless of his or her health insurance status, can receive urgent medical treatment. Article No. 7 of this Act provides for the possibility of access to urgent treatment for various groups of people, including people of unknown residence, foreigners from the states that have not signed a bilateral treaty with Slovenia, and all foreigners and citizens of Slovenia with permanent residence abroad; in addition, it provides that the Republic of Slovenia must assure that financial means directly from the state budget are intended for urgent treatment of those who are temporarily staying in or traveling through Slovenia and are unable to cover the costs of medical treatment. The Article also mentions other persons who are not covered by the compulsory health insurance system nor insured by a foreign health insurance provider/agency.

REFERENCES

Bauman, Z. 2005. "Freedom From, In and Through the State: T.H. Marshall's Trinity of Rights Revisited." *Theoria: A Journal of Social and Political Theory* 52(108): 13–27.

Becker, G. 2004. "Deadly Inequality in the Health Care 'Safety Net': Uninsured Ethnic Minorities' Struggle to Live with Life-Threatening Illnesses." *Medical Anthropology Quarterly* 18(2): 258–75.

Bon Gregorič, N., and J. Repič. 2016. "Introduction." In *Moving Places: Relations, Return and Belonging*, ed. Bon, N. and J. Repič, 1–21. New York: Berghahn Books.

Burcar, L. 2012. "Privatizacija in korporativizacija javne univerze [Privatization and corporatization of a public university]." *Šolsko polje* 23(3/4): 223–74.

Castro, A., and M. Singer, eds. 2004. *Unhealthy Health Policy: A Critical Anthropological Examination.* Lanham, MD: AltaMira Press.

Cresswell, T. 2006. *On the Move: Mobility in the Modern Western World.* New York: Routledge.

———. 2010. "Towards a Politics of Mobility." *Environment and Planning D: Society and Space* 28(1):17–31.

Dedič, J., V. Jalušič, and J. Zorn. 2003. *The Erased: Organized Innocence and the Politics of Exclusion.* Ljubljana: Peace Institute.

Fassin, D. 2004. "Social Illegitimacy as a Foundation of Health Inequality: How the Political Treatment of Immigrants Illuminates a French Paradox." In *Unhealthy Health*

Policy: A Critical Anthropological Examination, ed. A. Castro and M. Singer, 203–14. Lanham, MD: AltaMira Press.

Feldman, A. 1994. "Cultural Anesthesia: From Desert Storm to Rodney King." *American Ethnologist* 21(2): 404–18.

Horton, S. 2004. "Different Subjects: The Health Care System's Participation in the Differential Construction of the Cultural Citizenship of Cuban Refugees and Mexican Immigrants." *Medical Anthropology Quarterly* 18(4): 472–89.

Huysmans, J. 2000. "The Europan Union and the Securitisation of Migration." *Journal of Common Market Studies* 38(5): 751–77.

Huysmans, J. 2006. *The Politics of Insecurity: Fear, Migration and Asylum in the EU.* London: Routledge.

Inda, J. 2006. *Targeting Immigrants: Government, Technology, and Ethics.* Malden, MA: Blackwell.

Jazbinšek, S., and U. Lipovec Čebron. 2016. Focus group report – Slovenia. "Access to Health Care Services: Supporting Member States to Respond to the Health Needs of Asylum Seekers and Refugees." Unpublished report.

Kersnik, J. 2001. "Determinants of Customer Satisfaction with the Health Care System, with the Possibility to Choose a Personal Physician and with a Family Doctor in a Transition Country." *Health Policy* 57(2): 155–64.

Khan, N. 2016. "Immobility." In *Keywords of Mobility: Critical Engagements,* ed. N. B. Salazar and K. Jayaram, 93–112. New York: Berghahn Books.

Kogovšek, N., and B. Petkovič, eds. 2010. *The Scars of Erasure: A Contribution to the Critical Understanding of the Erasure of People from the Register of Permanent Residents of the Republic of Slovenia.* Ljubljana: Peace Institute.

Leskošek, V. 2013. "Vpliv paradigmatskih sprememb [The impact of paradigmatic changes]." In *Revščina zaposlenih* [Poverty of employees], ed. V. Leskošek, S. Smolej, L. Rihter, R. Boškovič, B. Kresal, and M. Breznik, 149–70. Ljubljana: Sophia.

———. "Migracije in dostop do socialnih pravic v EU in Sloveniji [Migration and access to social rights in the EU and Slovenia]." *Dve domovini/Two Homelands* 43: 91–102.

Leskošek, V., S. Smolej, L. Rihter, R. Boškovič, B. Kresal, and M. Breznik. 2013. "Sklep [Conclusion]." In *Revščina zaposlenih* [Poverty of employees], ed. V. Leskošek, S. Smolej, L. Rihter, R. Boškovič, B. Kresal, and M. Breznik, 201–6. Ljubljana: Sophia.

Lipovec Čebron, U. 2010. "The Construction of a Health Uninsurant: People without Medical Citizenship as Seen by Some Slovene Health Workers." *Studia ethnologica croatica* 22(1): 187–212.

———. 2011a. "Izbrisani prebivalci brez zdravstvenega državljanstva: medicinskoantropološka študija [Erased residents without medical citizenship: A medical anthropological study]." PhD dissertation. University of Ljubljana.

———. 2011b. "Reformiranje zdravstvenega sistema Slovenije: med 'lustracijskimi' in 'jugonostalgičnimi' težnjami [Reforming Slovenia's health system: Between "Yugonostalgia" and "lustration"]." *Etnolog* 21: 179–201.

Lipovec Čebron U., M. Svetel, and S. Pistotnik. 2015. "Zdravstveno marginalizirane skupine: prepreke, ovire, nepremostljivi zidovi do zdravja [Health marginalized groups: Obstacles and insurmountable walls to health]." Unpublished report. Together for Health, National Institute of Public Health, Slovenia.

Majcen, B., and M. Čok. 2014. "Ocena dolgoročne javno finančne vzdržnosti zdravstvenega sistema in možnih virov financiranja [Assessing the long-term fiscal sustainability of the health system and possible sources of financing]." Unpublished report. Retrieved 20 April 2016 from https://www.zav-zdruzenje.si/wp-content/uploads/2017/11/Ocena-dolgoro%C4%8Dne-javno-finan%C4%8Dne-vzdr%C5%BEljivosti-zdravstvenega-sistema-in-mo%C5%BEnih-virov-financiranja.pdf.

Markota, M., and T. Albreht. 2001. "Slovenian Experience on Health Insurance (Re)introduction." Croatian Medical Journal 42(1): 18–23.

Markota, M., I. Švab, K. Saražin Klemenčič, and T. Albreht. 1999. "Slovenian Experience on Health Care Reform." *Croatian Medical Journal* 40(2): 190–94.

Slovenia. Ministry of the Interior. 2015. "Migracije v številkah [Migration in numbers]." Retrieved 1 September 2016 from http://www.vlada.si/fileadmin/dokumenti/si/projekti/2015/begunci/160202_migranti.pdf.

MIPEX. 2015. "MIPEX—Country Report for EQUI-HEALTH." Brussels: International Organisation for Migration. Retrieved 10 July 2016 from http://www.mipex.eu/.

MSU and Akademska solidarnost. 2012. "Manifest proti privatizaciji visokega šolstva [A manifesto against the privatization of higher education]." Unpublished paper.

Ministry of Labour, Family, Social Affairs and Equal Opportunities. 2014. "Nacionalno socialno poročilo [National Social Report] (30.6.2013–1.7.2014)." Ljubljana: Ministry of Labour, Family, Social Affairs and Equal Opportunities. .

Mirovni inštitut. 2015. "Javno pismo Mirovnega inštituta [Public letter from the Peace Institute]." Press release, 6 November. Retrieved 12 April 2016 from http://www.mirovni-institut.si/javno-pismo-mirovnega-instituta/.

Peck, J. 2001. *Workfare States.* New York: Guilford Press.

Pistotnik, S. 2010. "The Erasure as a Testing Ground for European Migration Policies, or 'Pardon Me, but Your Regulations Have Erased My Status'." In *The Scars of Erasure: A Contribution to the Critical Understanding of the Erasure of People from the Register of Permanent Residents of the Republic of Slovenia,* ed. N. Kogovšek and B. Petkovič, 53–78. Ljubljana: Peace Institut.

Pistotnik, S., and U. Lipovec Čebron. 2015. "Predlogi sistemskih ukrepov za lažji dostop do zdravstvenega zavarovanja in do zdravstvenega varstva za odrinjene skupine [Proposals for systemic measures to facilitate access to health insurance and healthcare for marginalized persons]." Unpublished report. Together for Health, National Institute of Public Health, Slovenia.

Pravila obveznega zdravstvenega zavarovanja. 2003. "Pravila obveznega zdravstvenega zavarovanja [Compulsory Health Insurance Rules]." Uradni list RS 30/2003. Retrieved 5 June 2016 from http://www.pisrs.si/Pis.web/pregledPredpisa?id=DRUG1658.

Rajgelj, B. 2012. "Vpliv delovnopravnega, državljanskega in družinskopravnega statusa na neenako obravnavo v zdravstvenem zavarovanju [Impact of labor, citizenship and family status on unequal treatment in health insurance]." *Zdravstveno Varstvo* 51: 43–52.

Sheller, M., and J. Urry. 2006. "The New Mobilities Paradigm." *Environment and Planning A: Economy and Space* 38(2): 207–26.

Slovenia. Ministry of Health. 2010a. "Navodilo a sprejem pacientov v zdravstveno obravnavo v ambulantah nujne medicinske pomoči oziroma v sprejemnih ambulantah v bolnišnicah ter za obračun opravljenega dela [Admission instructions for outpatients' departments and hospitals in case of urgent medical treatment and financial assessment of medical services] ." Ljubljana: Ministry of Health.

Slovenia. Ministry of Health. 2010b. "Popravek Navodil za sprejem pacientov v zdravstveno obravnavo v ambulantah nujne medicinske pomoči oziroma v sprejemnih ambulantah v bolnišnicah ter za obračun opravljenega dela [Amendments to admission instructions for outpatients' departments and hospitals in case of urgent medical treatment and financial assessment of medical services]." Ljubljana: Ministry of Health.

Ticktin, M. 2006. "Where Ethics and Politics Meet: The Violence of Humanitarianism in France." *American Ethnologist* 33(1): 33–49.

Toth, M. 2003. *Zdravje, zdravstveno varstvo, zdravstveno zavarovanje* [Health, healthcare, health insurance]. Ljubljana: Zavod za zdravstveno zavarovanje Slovenije.

Tuccillo Castaldo, I. 2008. "Immobilized Citizenship." In *Once upon an Erasure: From Citizens to Illegal Residents in the Republic of Slovenia,* ed. J. Zorn and U. Lipovec Čebron. Special issue, *Časopis za kritiko znanosti* 35(228): 139–47.

Ustava Republike Slovenije. 1991. "Ustava Republike Slovenije [Constitution of the Republic of Slovenia]." Retrieved 1 March 2016 from http://www.pisrs.si/Pis.web/pregledPredpisa?id=USTA1.

Verlič-Christensen, B. 2002. *Evropa v precepu med svobodo in omejitvami migracij* [Europe amid freedom and restrictions on migration]. Ljubljana: Faculty of Social Sciences.

Walters, W. 2004. "Secure Borders, Safe Haven, Domopolitics." *Citizenship Studies* 8(3): 237–60.

Zakon o zdravstvenem varstvu in zdravstvenem zavarovanju (ZZVZZ-UPB3). 2006. "Zakono zdravstvenem varstvu in zdravstvenem zavarovanju (uradno prečiščeno besedilo) [Health Care and Health Insurance Act]." Uradni list RS, 72/2006. Retrieved 2 March 2016 from http://www.pisrs.si/Pis.web/pregledPredpisa?id=ZAK O213.

Zorn, J. 2010. "Registered as Workers, Erased as Non-Slovenes: The Transition Period from the Perspective of the Erased People." In *The Scars of Erasure: A Contribution to the Critical Understanding of the Erasure of People from the Register of Permanent Residents of the Republic of Slovenia,* ed. N. Kogovšek and B. Petkovič, 19–78. Ljubljana: Peace Institut.

Zorn, J. and U. Lipovec Čebron, eds. 2007. *Once upon an Erasure: From Citizens to Illegal Residents in the Republic of Slovenia.* Special issue, *Časopis za kritiko znanosti* 35(228).

PART II

The Effect of Imagination on Mobility as a Resource in the Search for Care and Caring

Anne E. Pfister

> People carry within their imaginations, memories and associated emotions that intersect both with the outward markers and physical baggage they bear and with the places they encounter.
>
> —Jennifer D. Adams, "Embodied Travel"

People's inner mobilities represent a confluence of emotion, memory, understanding, and imagination, and these internal phenomena continually interact with movement and place to shape mobility experience. Humans and other tangibles are in near-constant motion. The research featured in this section highlights external movements that serve as an entryway for studying people's inner mobility. Through direct observation, we perceive certain kinds of human mobility. People move about and carry things with them and these flows appear to be relatively straightforward. Physical mobility—especially movement of bodies and goods—are observable and traceable because this movement takes place externally. However, the chapters in this section focus on a more elusive form of mobility: the internal phenomena that accompany and personify those movements. These phenomena, including thought processes, emotions, and memories, are what Lean et al.

(2014: 9) refer to as "unique experiential baggage." Together, the chapters in this section expose the inner negotiations people engage as they consider and employ mobility as a resource in their search for care and caring.

The inner mobilities that characterize the unifying theme of this section take shape differently for the populations considered. In the first two chapters, narratives play a central role in understanding the imaginaries of participants and "convey the effort to make sense of the past from the perspective of the present" (Garro 2000: 71). Pfister and Vindrola-Padros focus on movement through stages of understanding and interpreting deaf diagnoses. At the heart of this chapter are participants' narratives of how they adapted to life with deaf offspring. As families of deaf children traveled around Mexico City seeking medical and educational options, parental reformulation of identity emerged. Speier's research follows a similar inquiry trajectory by focusing on the motivations of young Czech women who donate their eggs to fertilization clinics. The narrative accounts of young egg donors, like those of parents of deaf children, serve as what Garro (2000: 70) refers to as "retrospective assessments" in which participants "[draw] on their experiences and knowledge to link the past with present concerns and future possibilities." This chapter reveals the women's desires for status mobility—movement through financial, educational, health, and even moral statuses—as they use narrative reflection to contemplate and justify their choice to donate genetic material. We glimpse the internal mobility of the participants through their narratives that connect memory and experience with meaning and personal agency.

Finally, Plotnikova describes the migratory patterns of a mobile healthcare workforce with a particular focus on the policies aimed at regulating the mobility of healthcare workers. Yet, by drawing our attention to the outcomes that healthcare workers *imagine* will result from their movements, we are able to speculate about the motivations of these populations. Furthermore, by recognizing the importance of the imaginaries of these workers, we see how the policies Plotnikova outlines do not necessarily account for these less visible, internal, dynamic—and vitally important—factors affecting their decisions to migrate for work.

Together, the chapters in this section ask: *What role does imagination play as people conceptualize mobility options for care and caring?* Among Mexican families of deaf children, Pfister and Vindrola-Padros suggest, mobility allows parents of deaf children to evolve as they reconceptualize their children's condition and then modify their roles as caregivers. As these families physically move in and around Mexico City, they also move through understandings of deafness and disability, which in turn reshapes their identities. Speier's research suggests that young Czech women who participated in the reproductive travel industry were not only financially motivated, but also lured by how that flexible income would help them meet other, imagined goals. The women's narratives describe the kinds of mobility (e.g., status, income) they imagined and help us better understand the personal motivations propelling the physical movement of genetic and reproductive material. Plotnikova's analysis of policies attempting to regulate healthcare worker mobility reminds us that imaginaries of travel are distinctive and culturally situated. Yet, we are reminded that the slower-moving and less dynamic policies pertaining to migrating workforces do not address (nor adequately regulate) this ever-changing internal and external movement. Together, these chapters remind us that we cannot parse the "imaginaries" of travel from other, more obvious, external mobility forms.

Discussion Questions

In reading through the chapters in this section, it may be useful to keep the following questions in mind:

1. How does imagination affect how people conceive of mobility as a healthcare resource? Are there other aspects of imagination that affect mobility that are not mentioned in these chapters?
2. What are the methodological issues involved in accessing "imaginaries of travel"? How might the issues discussed in this section be addressed in other research contexts?
3. Plotnikova's research reveals gaps in policies pertaining to healthcare worker mobility. What kinds of changes in policies might address the discrepancies revealed throughout this section?

REFERENCES

Adams, J. 2014. "Embodied Travel: In Search of the Caribbean Self in Tropical Places and Spaces." In *Travel and Imagination,* ed. G. Lean, E. Waterton, and R. Staiff, 25–37. London, UK: Routledge.

Garro, L. 2000. "Cultural Knowledge as a Resource in Illness Narratives: Remembering through Accounts of Illness." In *Narrative and the Cultural Construction of Illness and Healing,* ed. C. Mattingly and L. Garro, 70–88. Berkeley, CA: University of California Press.

Lean et al. 2014. "Reimagining Travel and Imagination." In *Travel and Imagination,* ed. G. Lean, R. Staiff and E. Waterton, 9–22. London, UK: Routledge.

CHAPTER 4

Fluid and Mobile Identities

Travel, Imaginaries, and Caregiving Practices among Families of Deaf Children in Mexico City

Anne E. Pfister and Cecilia Vindrola-Padros

Instituto Pedagógico para Problemas de Lenguaje (IPPLIAP) is a deaf school in Colonia San Juan Mixcoac where Pfister conducted fieldwork from 2012 to 2013.[1] Mixcoac, as it is colloquially known, is in central Mexico City and is the childhood home of Octavio Paz, Mexican author, poet, and winner of the 1990 Nobel Prize for literature. Romanticized as an independent village during Paz's youth, Mixcoac, located approximately six miles southwest of the capital's historical center, is now a fully incorporated Mexico City *colonia* (neighborhood). Mixcoac is understood to be a solidly middle-class neighborhood, and IPPLIAP was located on a quiet, residential street near two other schools. Nonetheless, Mixcoac is not exempt from Mexico City's urban bustle; a newly expanded two-point metro transfer station was just three blocks from the school, and major traffic corridors bounded the neighborhood on all sides.

Like many of the students who attended IPPLIAP, I used public transportation, including the city's vast metro system, to travel between the school and my apartment located in a different Mexico City neighborhood. My commute was relatively short, especially compared to the average commute time for IPPLIAP families, many of whom traveled over two hours to school each morning. Walking from IPPLIAP to the metro station one afternoon,

I recognized an adolescent boy whom I confirmed was an IPPLIAP student by his school uniform. He walked with another young woman who did not appear to be an IPPLIAP student, yet seemed too young to be the boy's mother. I walked behind them and noticed how she walked a few paces ahead of him; I also noticed that they were not engaged in any kind of dialogue as they walked. During busier weekday commute times, metro authorities reserve the front cars of each train for women and children by creating guarded barricades men are not permitted to pass. The woman and boy headed through the barricade to those reserved trains, and since I was traveling in the same direction, I followed them. We boarded a relatively empty passenger car and I sat near the young man, who seated himself at a conspicuous distance from the young woman. He was tall and lean, crouched in his seat with his head tilted back against the seat. He looked quietly out the train window toward the dark tunnel of underground cave through which we would soon travel.

As we began to move, I tapped the boy's shoulder and made the Mexican sign for *hola* (hi) in *Lengua de Señas Mexicana* (Mexican Sign Language, or LSM). Both the boy and the young woman turned toward me, and initially, each seemed surprised to see me using LSM. After a brief moment, the boy quickly signed that he recognized me from IPPLIAP. We then introduced ourselves by finger-spelling our names and sharing our sign names. I used LSM to greet the young woman, but she told me in spoken Spanish, and through shy laughter, that she did not use sign language. Adrián,[2] the young man who attended IPPLIAP, was deaf and thus could not hear my brief oral exchange with his traveling partner. He tapped my shoulder to get my attention again, explaining to me in sign language that she was his cousin, she was hearing, and she did not use sign language. In the few minutes since our introduction, Adrián had quickly become social and animated. It was clear he wanted to converse as he darted from topic to topic as though we were old friends. As our conversation slowed and my stop approached, I asked him where they lived. He said they lived about an hour north, using a sign for a *colonia* with which I was unfamiliar (by some estimates, there are 350 *colonias* that constitute greater Mexico City, explaining why the city and surrounding area is sometimes referred to as a megalopolis). When Adrián recognized in my face that I was unfamiliar with his *colonia,* he pointed to the icon for the metro stop where they would eventually change trains, made the sign for it, and then used a series of signs to describe their journey: change, metro, bus, walk, ending with an emphatic *lejos* (far).

In these few minutes, I gathered valuable insight on the arduous urban trek Adrián and his cousin embarked upon each day. Through my observations, I surmised that their travels were not leisurely; vigilance and partnership were imperatives. Even as they might have appeared tired or aloof,

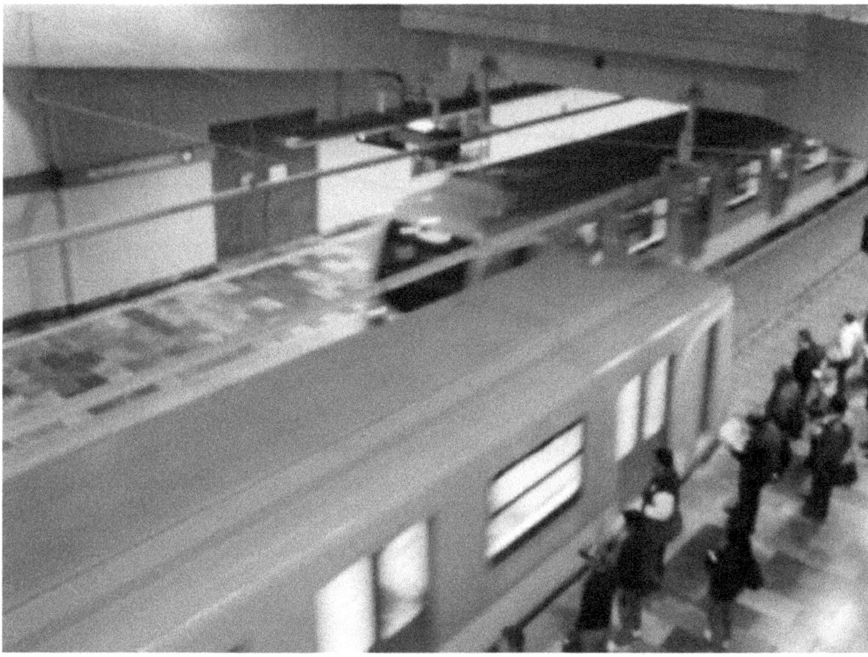

Figure 4.1 Image of the Mexico City Metro taken by Leo, an IPPLIAP student, during his commute to school. Photo courtesy of Leo (not a pseudonym, but the family surname of this participant is purposefully omitted).

they were wary of approaching strangers, monitoring the metro stops they passed along the way, and managing a multitude of other stimuli on Mexico City's crowded metro cars, streets, and tunnels. I also sensed an emotional burden—specifically, the cousin's sense of obligation. I imagined that chaperoning her deaf cousin across the city was a chore that she did when another responsible family member was not able to. I recognized how this might evoke something akin to resentment, even among the most dutiful and selfless of adolescent girls. Finally, while Adrián and his cousin moved together among countless other travelers, each of them seemed to travel in relative isolation. They were mostly anonymous among millions of strangers, and the language barrier between them would have made meaningful social exchange between them scant.

Care-Related Travel among Families with Deaf Children

Adrián and his cousin are one example of many family combinations who traveled to IPPLIAP so deaf children could experience sign-based education during the time this ethnography was conducted. Various forms of travel were time commitments that impinged upon any number of other endeavors, such as work, study, domestic chores, other familial duties, and rest. Time was chief among the many sacrifices families made to ensure their children could attend IPPLIAP. And yet, travel to IPPLIAP was, in many ways, relatively easy when compared to the earlier journeys these families made while seeking information and assistance for their deaf children, like those described later in this chapter. As the narratives of these families reveal, most initially found themselves traveling from one ineffective service to another in search of relevant information and assistance. The families featured in this chapter were among the rare few that found (and chose) a specialized deaf education at IPPLIAP. By the time these families found IPPLIAP, trial and error had revealed a promising, yet previously unimaginable, goal for their deaf children: sign language.

Not all journeys are the same. The purpose of travel, the circumstances, the people involved in travel, the conditions of the journey, and a myriad of other factors all play a role in shaping travel experiences. These factors also have an impact on travelers' process of identity construction. This chapter focuses on a relatively unique type of travel: the journeys endured by families seeking care for their deaf children. It draws from the experiences of families documented in an ethnographic study in Mexico where hearing parents traveled into and around areas of Mexico City to seek information about deafness and services for their deaf children. This chapter examines the fluid and multidimensional nature of identity among these families as they traveled. It examines identity formation as an inherently social process in which the collective and individual identity "are both produced, reproduced and changed" and are constantly undergoing transformational processes (Jenkins 1996: 19). The analysis of participants' narration of travel allows us to gain insight into specific aspects of the experience of families in motion as well as the role travel itself plays in processes of identity construction.

The discovery of children's deafness created a sense of disruption in the biographies of families, especially parents. The sense of normalcy in their family life became unsettled, which in turn spurned transformations in the way they saw their children and understood their role as parents and caregivers. In light of these exceptional circumstances, hearing parents found that one of the things they could do for their children was to make their best effort to secure the best type of care. The best care—a concept that was, in and of itself, dynamic for these families—was understood to be in Mexico City, and more specifically at IPPLIAP. Travel in and around Mexico City for many families meant enduring long and expensive trips, combining different forms of travel, spending time away from other family members, dealing with potentially unsafe surroundings, and encountering information that was often incomplete, conflicting, or difficult to access. Parents, while in a state of movement, interpreted and re-evaluated their understandings of the act of parenting. Their concepts of "care giving" changed and their identities were similarly dynamic.

Using families' narratives of travel and shifting identify as windows into their experience, this chapter closely examines the relationship between identity, care, and movement within families' social worlds. With a particular focus on the expectations of "care" in parenting, the authors frame identity formation as a product of socialization and re-socialization—understood in this chapter as social practices whereby people interpret and internalize the expectations by which they are to live. Travel for the purpose of obtaining care for deaf children can be used as a tangible analytic vehicle for understanding shifting parental roles and identities. The authors suggest that travel, when conceived of as an act or endeavor employed by the traveler, has the power to change one's perceptions of self and others. Journeys are times when travelers are able to explore potential identity transformations; identities are explored through direct experience during the journey and, importantly, through the process of narrating their journey to others. As this chapter demonstrates, families experienced various types of movement, which included (1) physical movement in search of information and services for their deaf children and (2) movement through identities. Through these different layers of movement, many hearing family members came to understand themselves as part of a "deaf family," something they had not previously imagined.

The Social Construction of Identity

We use an anthropological approach to understand the process of identity construction through movement in the particular circumstance of seeking care for deaf children, reminding us that "identity is a concept that figuratively combines the intimate or personal world with the collective space of cultural forms and social relations" (Holland et al. 1998: 5). Psychology has traditionally focused on the self and internalized attributes associated with identity. Identity is conceived of as something acquired in childhood that continues to develop, "[making] a human being a person and an acting individual" (Sökefeld 1999: 417). In contrast, anthropological perspectives seek identity through group affiliations, with a focus on the processes that take place between people and their social environments (Holland et al. 1998; Reynolds Whyte 2009). Baumeister (1986: 20) suggests identity is "any valid answer to the question 'Who are you?'" The framing of this question, the multitude of responses, and how these understandings change in time and place are of central importance to this ethnographic endeavor.

Anthropologists focus on two salient characteristics of identity: plurality and process. This holistic focus allows for the investigation of identity within dynamic contexts. Framed this way, authors conceptualize multiple identities (Galvin 2005; Ladd 2003; Leigh et al. 1998; Ochs 1993), preferred identities (Galvin 2005), the complexity and fluidity of identity (Ahmad et al. 2002; Breivik 2005; Corker 1998; Leigh 2008; LeMaster 2003; Skelton and Valentine 2003; Sökefeld 1999), intersectionality of identities (Valentine 2007) and the situational, negotiated, improvisational, and conflicting components of identity (Holland et al. 1998; Sökefeld 1999; Woodward 1997). Holland et al. (1998) develop "a picture of identity in practice." Intrigued by the improvisations people create in their everyday lives, they describe what occurs "when our past, brought to the present as habitus, meets with a particular combination of circumstances and conditions for which we have no set response" (pp. 17–18).

Disability and Identity: Biographical Disruption

The study of narrative construction and performance has provided valuable insight into processes of identity (re)formation (Bamberg 2012; Brockmeier and Carbaugh 2001; Frank 2012; Garro and Mattingly 2000; Holstein and Gubrium 2000). As Bamberg (2012: 102) indicates, "speakers, when making events (past, present, or fictitious) relevant for the here-and-now of speaking/listening activities, reveal aspects of who they are—they engage in identity claims with regard to how they would like to come across as well as in terms of potential answers to the who-am-I question." The construction of identity narratives is a collective and ongoing process involving the narrator, as well as the audience (or expected audience), and the context in which the story is told. Stories are told for a reason, and in the case of stories containing descriptions of the self, they reveal important details regarding how the narrators see themselves, the role they play—or are expected to play—in specific circumstances, and the ways in which they make sense of the world around them (Vindrola-Padros and Brage 2017).

Not all events are experienced or told in the same way. For example, the diagnosis of a disability is a significant, life-changing event for many families (Grant, Nolan, and Keady 2003). Such life events may cause "biographical disruption" (Bury 1982), a break in normal social routines and the "turning upside down" of daily life, potentially producing drastic changes in processes of identity construction (Kaufman 1988; Williams 1984). As Grant and colleagues (2003: 346) have explained, changes occur when "families become aware that they have become or are about to be responsible for the care of a child with disabilities." In this chapter, we look at these salient moments in the lives of Mexican families as biographical disruption.

The concept of biographical disruption has been used in previous analyses of parents' narratives of their child's disability to account for changes in their parental identity. Changes are often interpreted or experienced as the intensification of their parental role, which is manifested by their greater proximity to and focus on the special needs of the child (Chamberlayne and King 1997; Young et al. 2002). However, as Wilson (2007) has argued, in many ways, not only do the parents experience identity changes as a form of biographical disruption, but many also undergo a process of biographical reinforcement. In other words, a child's deaf diagnosis may act as the impetus for all of the subsequent actions recognized as part of their parental role, including the new duties and responsibilities associated with that role (see also Carricaburu and Pierret 1995). A continuously transforming parental identity and sense of self adapts to incorporate their child's diagnosis and need for specialized care. In effect, adapting to these new circumstances becomes part of parents' "biographical work" (Faircloth et al. 2004; Grant et al. 2003; Todd and Jones 2005). Furthermore, other factors taking place around the time of diagnosis, and in parents' search for care for their children, might play a more significant role in their self-definition as parents and thus feature more prominently in their personal narratives (for examples in different contexts, see Adamson and Donovan 2005; Ciambrone 2001; Pound, Gompertz, and Ebrahim 1998; Young et al. 2002). For the participants in this study, the need to travel to search for information and services for deaf children was a noticeable factor affecting both the personal narratives and the identities these narratives reveal.

Travel, Identity, and the Imaginary

Studies on the experiences of travelers underscore how the act of traveling (both physical and in the imaginary) is a process imbued with meaning. The imagination, understood as "dreams, make-believe, fantasy, memory and remembering, perception, the 'mind's eye', understanding, world-views, learning, story-telling" (Lean, Staiff, and Waterton 2014: 12), creates particular expectations and experiences of travel (Lean Staiff, and Waterton 2014; Salazar 2012). Travel can function as a rite of passage, a transition between different life stages (White and White 2004). It can be used to search for something that is missing from daily life, as a source of enrichment or escape, or as a way to find a better life for oneself or one's family (Ateljevic and Doorne 2000; Lanfrant 1995). Travel experiences, both lived and told, have the potential to produce profound changes in the identities of travelers. Stories about journeys become part of what Desforges (2000) calls imaged performances of the self, where travelers are able to think about and portray themselves in different ways (White and White 2004). During the construction of stories depicting journeys, the narrators (in this case, the travelers) choose to highlight particular aspects of the journeys, while giving other components less importance or even leaving them untold (White and White 2004). Often, aspects told and highlighted are selected to create a particular image of the traveler that responds to the specific time and context in which the story is performed.

Some researchers suggest "narrative is one of the most powerful tools that humans possess for organizing and interpreting experience" (Van Deusen-Phillips et al. 2001: 311) and narrative-based approaches have been recognized as helping make participants' knowledge relevant (Lende and Lachiondo 2009). A closer look at the travel experiences of families of deaf children points to the wide range of factors at play during travel. Of particular interest for this chapter is how some experiences have a profound impact on identity and caregiving. This perspective allows us to expand our understanding of travel beyond the physical act of movement, to encompass a broader range of mobilities, including those that take place in the mind (Lean et al. 2014).

Research Context

One of the authors conducted research among mostly hearing families of deaf children in central Mexico City (Pfister 2015). One of the world's most densely populated cities, Mexico City includes the bustling *Distrito Federal* (federal district) and the surrounding urban sprawl that, together, boasted over nineteen million residents as of July 2013 (CIA 2014). The predominant approach to deafness in Mexico City is a distinctly medicalized stance (Pfister 2015). The medicalized construction of deafness, also referred to as the infirmity or pathological model, is a paradigm that underscores the physiological state of deafness by understanding it as something to be cured, and often presents deaf people as disabled. By contrast, proponents of a deaf cultural identity model emphasize the shared experience, language, and culture in deaf communities and do not view deafness as a disability (Corker 1998; Ladd 2005; Lane 1995; Phillips 1996; Ramsey and Noriega 2001; Rosen 2003). Worldwide, generally accepted estimates claim that upwards of 90 percent of deaf children are born to hearing parents (Mitchell and Karchmer 2004); the majority of deaf children in this study were born to hearing families thus following that trend (Pfister 2015).

Discovering Deafness

At the time of this research, IPPLIAP (Pfister's primary research site) was the only sign language–based Mexican institution offering a nationally recognized certificate of primary education to its graduates. IPPLIAP taught LSM alongside written Spanish. IPPLIAP served approximately 115 students during the time of this research and was one of only three small, semiprivate schools in Mexico City. For these reasons and more, families traveled from distant parts of Mexico City so their deaf children could take advantage of this rare educational opportunity. Because there were so few accessible educational options for deaf children in Mexico, families made tremendous time sacrifices in order to bring their children to IPPLIAP. Though the average commute time to IPPLIAP was just over two hours each way, many parents, including Eulalia (below), traveled more than six hours daily accompanying their children on public transportation to the school.

Many mothers, like Eulalia, waited on campus while their children were in school, often volunteering around the school to offset tuition costs. Pfister met families on campus, including through her participation in IPPLIAP-sponsored events like LSM classes and educational advisory board meetings. The vast majority of the hearing family participants in this study did not have experience with deafness prior to their child's diagnosis, did not have contact with a deaf community, and were unfamiliar with sign language when they discovered their child's deafness. Eulalia's identical twin daughters, both deaf, attended IPPLIAP. The twins—or *las gemelas,* as they were known by their family and acquaintances—were deafened at birth. During a one-on-one interview, Pfister asked Eulalia what she knew about deafness at the time she discovered her daughters' deafness. She replied:

> Well, when they gave me the diagnosis, I didn't know anything. So, I felt quite alienated. And then, they told me later that with the hearing aids the girls would recuperate their hearing 80 percent, I said, "What a miracle!" . . . I mean, I was a person who didn't really know about these kinds of things. So, of course, I didn't realize it wasn't true until so much time had passed.

Concerned about their children's language development, and influenced by biomedical practitioners who advised against the use of sign language, Mexican hearing family participants, including Eulalia, experimented with biomedical interventions and enrolled their deaf children in intensive oral therapy (or speech therapy). As they operationalized "care" in an attempt to address their deaf children's language needs, Mexican hearing families' obligations transitioned in unanticipated ways—from naturalized language and socialization models to being caregivers in search of information and interventions. For these families, the "familiar" process of language socialization became "strange" in biomedical settings.

While advocates for sign language exist in Mexico, a distinctly medicalized stance toward deafness prevails. Advocates of an overtly medicalized approach to deafness seldom recognize opportunities to learn sign language or to integrate into a signing community as valid options for deaf children. Many families who navigated Mexico City's medical system encountered limited, perplexing, and often false information regarding deafness and sign language. Biomedical and therapeutic interventions tempted families with the idea that their child's deafness could be miraculously fixed through interventions such as hearing aids and cochlear implants (hearing aids amplify sound and cochlear implants are surgically implanted devices that stimulate the auditory nerve). One participant said it best when she said that hearing aids were marketed as though they worked like glasses: you just put them on and suddenly you can hear. Following encounters with medical practitioners in this context, parents often believed their children were sick, *descompuesto* (broken), and/or disabled. The comments of Ángel, whose eight-year-old son was deaf, reflected his internalization of the tenets of the Mexican medicalized model:

> I had the need to believe that my son was sick and that he could be cured. My wife also wanted to believe that, if her son was deaf, he could be cured. So, we continued down the track, doing what the doctors advised, but we didn't see results.

An important part of these families' journeys, and the resulting shift in their identities as parents of deaf children, was the act of accepting their child's deafness. As parents explained their own conceptual progression through narrative, they were also articulating how they began to see their earlier notions about "fixing" their deaf child as misguided. In other words, they recognized their own shifting perspectives on their roles. Here, Carmen relayed how she regularly encountered views that her deaf son could be "repaired":

> Even my mother, she still says, "It's because when the child *se componga* (is repaired), he will speak. I'm telling you." But, of course, I understand now it's not a matter of repairing him. This is how he is, and we have to accept it.

While many parent participants eventually came to realizations similar to Carmen's, most experienced a strong desire to find a "cure" for their children, particularly as they began their service-seeking journeys. Misconceptions about deafness and the ubiquity of biomedical interventions in Mexico fueled the desire among participants and medical personnel to "repair" deafness. The perceived validity and relevancy of biomedical approaches ebbed and flowed among participants as they encountered new environments and engaged with different kinds of information about deafness.

Navigating Mexico's Public Health System: Traveling to *el Hospital*

Mexican families' care-seeking journeys typically began in medical establishments where families consulted doctors for advice on coping with a child's deafness. At the *Instituto Nacional de Rehabilitación* (National Institute for Rehabilitation, or INR) and in other clinical settings, hearing family participants were confronted with specific ideas about deafness and disability. For example, doctors usually presented intensive speech therapy in tandem with medical interventions (see also Pfister 2017).

General practitioners and public health clinics were typically parents' first stops in their journeys. These early encounters with medical practitioners came at a time when parents were impressionable, as many were still reeling from the shock of diagnosis. Thus, early encounters set the tone for subsequent stages in their treatment-seeking journeys. Doctors and medical practitioners described deafness as a "disorder" and a "disability." Under this paradigm, deafness was a "problem" that required intervention to attempt to be "fixed" or "cured." In these early visits, doctors often referred participants to the INR. As the only national institute dedicated to speech and hearing disorders, the INR was heralded by public practitioners as the nexus of audiology and speech specialty, and it was the home of current technology that could determine a child's "precise" capacity for hearing through audiometric testing. People from all over the Republic of Mexico traveled to visit the INR, which was crowded and highly bureaucratic, with a decidedly hospital-like feel. Many hearing participants understood, at least initially, that a trip to the INR with their deaf child was essentially mandatory. Scores of ambulances parked out front; people with acute medical needs enter through the same doors as deaf children seeking speech therapy. One visit quickly reveals why many participants referred to the INR simply as *el hospital*.

The medical model of deafness is characterized by what Clough and Corbett (2000: 11) call "a *pathology of difference*" (emphasis in original). In Mexico and other contexts heavily influenced by the medical model, deafness is constructed as a disability, which underscores and pathologizes deaf children's difference (biological differences affecting hearing, but also linguistic differences as they relate to accessing language). Under medical models, disability becomes the "province of medicine [with a focus on] medical intervention [and] emphasis on 'abnormality', disorder, and limited function" (Brett 2002: 828). Accordingly, Mexican deaf children are separated from their peers, and the alleged deficiencies are tested for, measured, diagnosed, and sometimes treated in clinics like the INR.

Eunice claimed the long lines at the INR kept her from pursuing assistance there. She was not the only participant to express an opinion that time spent at the INR felt futile:

> They sent us to the institute, but there, just trying to get an appointment is a total mess. And then, it's only to find that the doctor is away at a conference, or is on vacation, or the like. The truth is, I just stopped going. . . . I never went back, that's the truth. For me, it was like a big waste, because later I was pregnant with another child and it just didn't seem worthwhile. . . . We would have to be there exactly on time and, if not, they wouldn't give us the appointment. And there we were running around. All the time. So [I just thought], well, no.

Dealing with Deceit and Misinformation

Mexican parents of deaf children complained of the public medical system's lack of a clear, systematic protocol for finding assistance for their children. This contributed to families' movement from place to place in search of information. Carmen's story echoes experiences heard from many parents who felt frustrated when they could not identify a stepwise path for successful navigation within the institute. Carmen used repetitive questioning in her narrative to illustrate how she felt that her concerns were not adequately addressed:

> We were with the doctors at the hospital when we actually realized that he didn't hear well, because they didn't tell us at first that our child had that problem (deafness). The medical professionals said, "well, he's going to need a hearing aid" and I asked, "okay, all right, where do I get them?' They responded, "no, well it's just that you have to go and find out if you can get them donated." So, I said, "but where?" They said, "go see if you can get them donated." So, I said, "but where?" They said, "go to the hospital." So, that's where we went.
>
> Then, at *el hospital* they said, "but you have to wait, you have to do this and that, and you have to be here in this course of therapy." I mean, really, they never told us, "you know what? You're going to have to go to this place, there they'll sell you a hearing aid, and that's what you need." Nothing. And then when one goes to actually get the hearing aid, that's also many times a real *engaño* [sham].

At the end of this passage, Carmen used the word *engaño* to summarize her experiences with the audiology professionals. The word, from the verb *engañar,* translates as "deceit," "fraud," or "hoax." Carmen hints at her disapproval of the medical establishment at the start of her narrative when she recalls the relatively late diagnosis of her son's deafness, at three years of age. Her repetitive questioning invokes the futility she felt in her search for information about deafness and echoes a perception among many parent participants. In the last sentence, she clearly states that she believes audiologists trick and betray their patients.

During the time surrounding diagnosis, deafness was still new to her and she had limited knowledge about this condition, like other parents. Carmen went on to express how she remembers feeling uneasy and alone in this new parenting role and suggested the value of finding others with similar experiences:

> Really, you aren't sure until you get to know other people. . . . [Pfister interrupts to ask, "more people with experience?"] More people with experience, yes. Because [medical personnel] keep telling us "do this or that" . . . but they never make clear what we should *really* do.

Carmen, like other family participants, felt alienated and intimidated in medical environments where she was isolated from others who were experiencing similar parenting struggles. She, like others, sought "insider" knowledge—in the form of networking and community building—among "more people with experience." This excerpt suggests she believed community (and socialization) could at least partially ameliorate her lack of confidence in the medical establishment.

Parents soon realized clinical settings were not the place to find either useful information on deafness or the support they sought. However, their travels into and around Mexico City eventually led them to a community of families with deaf children where information and resources were shared. The "experts" and shared repertoire they desired were found in a community that formed around a specialized deaf school, not at a hospital or clinic. This discovery—often accidental—was an important shift in families' journeys.

Changing the Destination

Parents soon realized for themselves that there is no cure for deafness, despite the promising-sounding treatment and intervention options that families of deaf children encounter. Deaf individuals have different capacities to perceive sound and different life histories, and these are just two factors affecting differential responses to interventions and therapy. When their deaf children did not conform to normative hearing standards, as biomedical practitioners offering interventions suggested they should, participants soon realized that these interventions offered unrealistic promises. Many deaf children and adults were unable to speak or fully access Spanish, despite their dedication and perseverance in oral therapy. Nearly all families in Pfister's study felt dismayed by the slow progress their children made in speech therapy, often referring to it as "time wasted."

A pivotal point for families with deaf children—at least for the participants in this study—was incorporation into a sign-based community of practice at IPPLIAP, a semiprivate, not-for-profit primary school. Due to the prevalence of medical professionals' advice that parents avoid sign language for their deaf children, many families did not actively seek deaf educational opportunities and deaf communities. Interviews with families revealed no one clear path leading families to IPPLIAP. For example, stigmatizing ideas surrounding sign language are common in Mexico—myths such as "sign language is for monkeys" are in wide circulation. Thus, many family members faced resistance from their spouses and other relatives who did not want their deaf children to learn sign language. Many participants initially felt that by exposing their children to signing, they were essentially going against "doctor's orders." As such, two themes emerged from interviews with regard to how participating families found IPPLIAP. Some described serendipitous encounters with families with deaf children at IPPLIAP. Often, these chance encounters happened on the metro, when a mother of a deaf child recognized a stranger with a deaf child, for example, and approached her to recommend IPPLIAP. A second theme involved families who heard about IPPLIAP and may have dismissed the idea early on. Later, many came to IPPLIAP, viewing it as a last resort when other interventions (therapy and hearing aids, for example) had failed their children.

The families who found IPPLIAP and sent their children to school there underwent an intense paradigmatic shift. As their children began to learn LSM, hearing parents witnessed profound changes in their deaf children's learning and behavior, which they often described as "incredible" and "a panorama" opening. The imagery evoked by the word "panorama" is useful for conceptualizing how sign language functioned to create the linguistic and social space necessary for language learning and inclusive socialization among deaf youth. Participants repeatedly expressed that their family's sacrifices were worthwhile in order to be able to send their deaf children to IPPLIAP. Ángel said,

> When my son began to learn LSM, another option suddenly appeared before me. Now, in signs, he calls me *papá*. So, in his hands, I see his

> voice, the voice that I'm never going to hear. I'm encouraged and it gives me peace because I always carried that pain of not being able to understand what he wanted.

As they watched their children learn and flourish at IPPLIAP, parents' and families' identities shifted—many began to think of themselves as "deaf families." As they met other families in the community, they happily spoke of the benefits of becoming "bilingual" and "bi-cultural." They referenced perks such as the ability to use sign language in crowded spaces where it was hard to hear. But, above all, they beamed when relaying the importance of the unity and contentment their children experienced as they were incorporated into a social world where they could participate fully.

Jorge, who described his son as a "parrot" who simply repeated things he learned in hospital-endorsed language therapy, described how LSM facilitated their son's Spanish acquisition. Jorge and his wife, Clara, indicated that their son was able to understand the meaning of words in Spanish through the simultaneous use of LSM. This also helped them teach him new concepts. Jorge said this about IPPLIAP:

> We realize now, after much time wasted, that we should have looked for an option like IPPLIAP earlier for our son. I mean, it's incredible, it's not just notable, it's *incredible* the change that our son underwent after only his first week here. (emphasis in original)

Like Jorge and Clara, most participants in this study considered themselves lucky to have had the opportunity to participate in the sign-based community of practice at IPPLIAP. Families also demonstrated awareness that they were among the minority of families with deaf children in Mexico who had access to a bilingual school for their children. Some family identities had shifted significantly—from parents who knew virtually nothing about deafness to parents who now thought of themselves as a "deaf family." For example, Patricia said,

> We are a deaf family. We use LSM, we all communicate that way, visually. And we have integrated into our son's culture. We are here at this school, we embrace it. And culturally, we are deaf.

Families acquired the experience of deafness as a shared identity through a time marked by persistent mobility. Though initially the concept of deafness was difficult for parents to understand and accept, they eventually discovered the deaf cultural concept for themselves. They eventually interpreted and cultivated this newfound concept as part of their parenting identities, essentially re-socializing themselves as parents. Upon integration into the community at IPPLIAP, parents realized that their own lived experiences of deafness contrasted sharply with the medicalized understandings of deafness they had encountered early on when deafness was depicted as "abnormality," "illness," and "disability." Often for the first time, they experienced conviviality with others who had similar experiences. In other words, families connected with one another intersubjectively at IPPLIAP; they experienced community interconnectivity based on mutual sharing and understanding of experience (Zlatev 2007). Intersubjective experience allowed these families the freedom to shed the fears, ideas, and identities associated with their pre-deaf lives and their early, unsettling experiences with deaf diagnoses. This intersubjective experience harkens Nichter's (2002: 82) recollection of "the work of culture," which "involves a reappraisal and reframing of troubles and negative emotions in terms of publicly accepted sets of meaning and symbols." IPPLIAP facilitated an environment that nurtured families and simultaneously transformed parent and family identities. Supported by this newly found comfort, families were able to still their movement and settle into the IPPLIAP community. They adapted and transformed their identities and adjusted to their new roles.

Conclusions

The authors of this chapter recognize that not all parents and medical practitioners view "disability" monolithically. Experiences with deafness and disability manifest differently among individuals, in institutions, and within families. Furthermore, we recognize that not all individuals perceive deafness as a disability and that context is important in interpretation and experience. Indeed, the goal of this chapter is to illustrate how parents' notions of deafness and disability are fluid and subject to change, even within rigid medicalized contexts. Furthermore, research among parents of children with disabilities reveals evidence that factors such as income, family support, and availability of time for parent-child interactions have measurable effects on parental stress in families with children with disabilities (Olson et al. 1999; Smith et al. 2001). Early research traditionally emphasized the negative impact of parenting deaf children, including shock, grief, sorrow and depression (Moses 1985) and chronic stress (Quittner et al. 1990). Yet these findings are tempered by studies revealing that parents of deaf children were not necessarily under more duress or less satisfied than parents of hearing children (Lederberg and Goldbach 2002; Meadow-Orlans 1994; Pipp-Siegel et al. 2001). Again, social support was an influential factor in parental satisfaction and stress in this study. In other words, the intensity of "biographical disruption" may correlate with perceived stress among participants, factors that were likely differential among families.

Nonetheless, the hearing families participating in this study often perceived deaf diagnoses initially as a "disability." Parents described unanticipated discoveries of deafness that created what participants described as a "shock." Thus, discovery of deafness disrupted parents' imaginaries of parenthood, and they realized that a different type of care—care that parents initially did not understand well—was now necessary for their child(ren). This study reveals narratives depicting how parents developed what Hunt (2000: 90) calls a "strategically revised identity." In the case of Mexican families in this study, travel to find the best care for their children was central to identity revision, and movement was evident in their narration of their lives. Identity revision—and the accompanying narratives—also allowed parents to relate to others with similar experiences, including people with whom they otherwise may never have previously associated. As they revised their identities and narrated their experiences, they simultaneously adapted to new roles and responsibilities as parents. Knowledge gained through experience and mobility allowed them to see themselves in a new light by incorporating "deafness" as part of their new identity.

Parents in this study experienced a gamut of emotions as they assimilated news of their child's deaf diagnosis; some described experiencing despair, denial, and isolation. But, after the initial shock subsided, parents realized they had to do something. In an attempt to interpret and understand their new caretaking roles, these families became mobile. Their movement was motivated by a quest for information and a desire to help their children, even though most did not have a particular destination in mind. As families embarked upon their journeys, they encountered different people, communities, and information. Travel was transitional and necessary during this time in their lives, but it was also a time in which these families connected socially in new ways. Through these new circles of socialization, they were freed from the isolation they had experienced surrounding the deaf diagnosis of their child(ren). Through physical movement, and movement through different identities, families came to terms with, assimilated, and interpreted information about deafness personally and through social interactions. Through this movement, they transitioned from feeling isolated (without community) to an identity they could not have imagined ("parents of deaf children" or even "deaf families").

The process of socialization and identity re-formation allowed them to experience intersubjective connections among other families who were experiencing similar unanticipated circumstances. The community of IPPLIAP formed around intersubjective familiarity, and this created a space where families were free to recreate their identities. As IPPLIAP emerged as a destination for these travelers, they were able to settle into this community and reflect upon their journeys through narrative. In sum, families interpreted deafness for themselves through movement and this was a fundamentally social process. Their narratives underscore how this movement and these processes act as space in which "priorities are (re-)established and social relationships revisited" (Nichter 2002: 101).

Contextual understandings of deafness and disability permeate the shifting responsibilities and identities of family members as "caretakers" and deaf children as the recipients of such care. This recalls Elinor Ochs's (1986) notion of children as socializers. In 1986, Ochs wrote, "Children are active socializers of others in their environment. Even infants and small children have a hand in socializing other members of their family into such roles as care-giver, parent, and sibling" (p. 2). At first blush, this statement may seem obvious. However, Ochs reminds us of something important: socialization is ongoing throughout the life course and, during this process, identities are continually constructed and re-constructed. The experiences of these families confirm that through the multidirectional and dialectical process of constructing and re-constructing identity, families navigate between identifying as parents of "sick" or "well" children, as parents of "able" or "disabled" children, as "care takers" and "care givers." Their stories remind us that children and adults continually interpret, negotiate, and internalize the expectations and identities attached to these roles.

Anne E. Pfister, PhD, is assistant professor of anthropology at the University of North Florida. Her research investigates how deaf youth and their families experience deafness in Mexico City by integrating sociocultural linguistic theory with biocultural medical anthropology analyses. Her project utilizes visual methods, including "photovoice," to actively engage participants as co-researchers. She has been involved with the Mexican deaf community for over ten years. Dr Pfister's research interests include disabilities studies, language socialization, and medicalization; her work has been published in *Ethos, Visual Anthropology Review, Behavioral and Brain Sciences, Collaborative Anthropologies,* and *Annals of Anthropological Practice.*

Cecilia Vindrola-Padros, PhD, is a research associate in the Department of Applied Health Research, University College London, UK. She is a medical anthropologist and has researched the experiences of children and families who relocate to access medical treatment. Recent publications on mobility include the book chapters "Children Seeking Health Care: International Perspectives on Children's Use of Mobility to Obtain Health Services" (with Ginger Johnson), in *Mobilities and Journeys: Geographies of Children and Young People* (Springer, 2017), and "Child Medical Travel in Argentina: Narratives of Family Separation and Moving Away from Home" (with Eugenia Brage), in *Children's Health and Wellbeing in Urban Environments* (Routledge, 2017).

NOTES

1. This introductory vignette is told from Pfister's first-person perspective. Analysis of these data is the work of both authors.
2. All of the names used in this chapter are the participants' names. Each gave explicit permission to use her name and image for research purposes during the informed consent process.

REFERENCES

Adamson, J., and J. Donovan. 2005. "'Normal Disruption': South Asian and African/ Caribbean Relatives Caring for an Older Family Member in the UK." *Social Science & Medicine* 60(1): 37–48.

Ahmad, Waqar I. U., Karl Atkin, and Lesley Jones. 2002. "Being Deaf and Being Other Things: Young Asian People Negotiating Identities." *Social Science & Medicine* 55(10): 1757–1769.

Ateljevic, I., and S. Doorne. 2000. "Tourism as an Escape: Long-Term Travellers in New Zealand." *Tourism Analysis* 5(2–4): 131–36.

Bamberg, M. 2012. "Narrative Practice and Identity Navigation." In *Varieties of Narrative Analysis*, ed. J. Holstein and J. Gubrium, 99–122. Los Angeles, CA: SAGE.

Baumeister, Roy F. 1986. *Identity: Cultural Change and the Struggle for Self.* Oxford and New York: Oxford University Press.

Breivik, Jan-Kåre. 2005. *Deaf Identities in the Making: Local Lives, Transnational Connections.* Washington, DC: Gallaudet University Press.

Brett, Jane. 2002. "The Experience of Disability from the Perspective of Parents of Children with Profound Impairment: Is it Time for an Alternative Model of Disability?" *Disability & Society* 17(7): 825–843.

Brockmeier, J., and D. Carbaugh. 2001. *Narrative and Identity: Studies in Autobiography, Self and Culture.* Amsterdam: John Benjamins.

Bury, M. 1982. "Chronic Illness as Biographical Disruption." *Sociology of Health & Illness* 4(2): 167–82.

Carricaburu, D., and J. Pierret. 1995. "From Biographical Disruption to Biographical Reinforcement: The Case of HIV-Positive Men." *Sociology of Health & Illness* 17(1): 65–88.

Chamberlayne, P., and A. King. 1997. "The Biographical Challenge of Caring." *Sociology of Health & Illness* 19(5): 601–21.

Ciambrone, D. 2001. "Illness and Other Assaults on Self: The Relative Impact of HIV/ AIDS on Women's Lives." *Sociology of Health & Illness* 23(4): 517–40.

Clough, Peter, and Jenny Corbett. 2000. *Theories of Inclusive Education: A Student's Guide.* London: Sage Publications Ltd.

Corker, Mairian. 1998. *Deaf and Disabled, Or Deafness Disabled? Towards a Human Rights Perspective.* Buckingham: Open University Press.

Desforges, L. 2000. "Traveling the World: Identity and Travel Biography." *Annals of Tourism Research* 27(4): 926–45.

Faircloth, C., C. Boylstein, M. Rittman, M. Young, and J. Gubrium. 2004. "Sudden Illness and Biographical Flow in Narratives of Stroke Recovery." *Sociology of Health & Illness* 26(2): 242–61.
Frank, A. 2012. "Practicing Dialogical Narrative Analysis." In *Varieties of Narrative Analysis,* ed. J. Holstein and J. Gubrium, 33–50. Los Angeles, CA: SAGE.
Galvin, Rose. 2005. "Researching the Disabled Identity: Contextualising the Identity Transformations Which Accompany the Onset of Impairment." *Sociology of Health Illness* 27(3): 393–413.
Garro, L., and C. Mattingly. 2000. "Narrative as Construct and Construction." In *Narrative and the Cultural Construction of Illness and Healing,* ed. C. Mattingly and L. Garro, 1–49. Berkeley, CA: University of California Press.
Grant, G., M. Nolan, and J. Keady. 2003. "Supporting Families over the Life Course: Mapping Temporality." *Journal of Intellectual Disability Research* 47(4/5): 342–51.
Holland, Dorothy C., William Jr Lachicotte, Carole Cain, and Debra Skinner.1998. *Identity and Agency in Cultural Worlds.* Cambridge, MA: Harvard University Press.
Holstein, J. A., and J. Gubrium. 2000. *The Self We Live By: Narrative Identity in a Postmodern World.* New York: Oxford University Press.
Hunt, L. 2000. "Strategic Suffering: Illness Narratives as Social Empowerment among Mexican Cancer Patients." In *Narrative and the Cultural Construction of Illness and Healing,* ed. C. Mattingly and L. Garro, 88–107. Berkeley, CA: University of California Press.
Jenkins, Richard. 1996. *Social Identity.* London: Routledge.
Kaufman, S. 1988. "Toward a Phenomenology of Boundaries in Medicine: Chronic Illness Experience in the Case of Stroke." *Medical Anthropology Quarterly* 2(4): 338–54.
Ladd, Paddy. 2005. "Deafhood: A Concept Stressing Possibilities, Not Deficits." *Scandinavian Journal of Public Health* 33(5): 12.
Ladd, Paddy. 2003. *Understanding Deaf Culture: In Search of Deafhood.* Clevedon and Buffalo, NY: Multilingual Matters.
Lane, Harlan.1995. Constructions of Deafness. *Disability & Society* 10(2): 171–190.
Lanfrant, M. 1995. "Introduction." In *International Tourism: Identity and change,* ed. M. Lanfrant, J. Allcock, and E. Bruner, 1–23. London: SAGE.
Lean, G., R. Staiff, and E. Waterton. 2014. "Reimagining Travel and Imagination." In *Travel and Imagination,* ed. G. Lean, R. Staiff, and E. Waterton, 9–24. New York: Routledge.
Lederberg, A. R. and T. Golbach. 2002. "Parenting Stress and Social Support in Hearing Mothers of Deaf and Hearing Children: A Longitudinal Study." *Journal of Deaf Studies and Deaf Education* 7 (4): 330–345.
Leigh, Irene W. 2008. "Who Am I? Deaf Identity Issues." In *Signs and Voices: Deaf Culture, Identity, Language and Arts,* ed. Kristin A. Lindgren, Doreen DeLuca and Donna Jo Napoli, 21–29. Washington, DC: Gallaudet University Press.
Leigh, Irene W., Alan L. Marcus, Patricia K. Dobosh, and Thomas E. Allen. 1998. "Deaf/Hearing Cultural Identity Paradigms: Modification of the Deaf Identity Development Scale." *Journal of Deaf Studies and Deaf Education* 3(4): 329–338.

LeMaster, Barbara. 2003. "School Language and Shifts in Irish Deaf Identity." In *Many Ways to Be Deaf: International Variation in Deaf Communities,* ed. Leila Frances Monaghan, 153–173. Washington, DC: Gallaudet University Press.

Lende, Daniel H., and Alicia Lachiondo. 2009. "Embodiment and Breast Cancer among African American Women." *Qualitative Health Research* 19(2): 216–228.

Meadow-Orlans, Kathryn P. 1994. "Stress, Support, and Deafness Perceptions of Infants' Mothers and Fathers." *Journal of Early Intervention* 18 (1): 91–102.

Mitchell, Ross E., and Michael A. Karchmer. 2004. "Chasing the Mythical Ten Percent: Parental Hearing Status of Deaf and Hard of Hearing Students in the United States." *Sign Language Studies* 4(2): 138.

Moses, K. L. 1985. "Infant Deafness and Parental Grief: Psychosocial Early Intervention." In *Education of the Hearing Impaired Child,* ed. F. Powell, T. Finitzo-Hieber, S. Friel-Patti, and D. Henderson, 86–102. San Diego, CA: College-Hill.

Ochs, Elinor, and Bambi B. Schieffelin. 1986. *Language Socialization Across Cultures.* Cambridge and New York: Cambridge University Press.

Ochs, Elinor. 1993. "Constructing Social Identity: A Language Socialization Perspective." *Research on Language and Social Interaction* 26(3): 287–306.

Olsen, Susanne Frost, Elaine Sorensen Marshall, Barbara L. Mandleco, Keith W. Allred, Tina Taylor Dyches, and Nancy Sansom. 1999. "Support, Communication, and Hardiness in Families with Children with Disabilities." *Journal of Family Nursing* 5 (3): 275–291.

Phillips, Barbara A. 1996. "Bringing Culture to the Forefront: Formulating Diagnostic Impressions of Deaf and Hard-of-Hearing People at Times of Medical Crisis." *Professional Psychology: Research and Practice* 27(2): 137.

Pipp-Siegel, S., A. L. Sedey, and C. Yoshinaga-Itano. 2002. "Predictors of Parental Stress in Mothers of Young Children with Hearing Loss." *Journal of Deaf Studies and Deaf Education* 7 (1): 1–17.

Pound, P., P. Gompertz, and S. Ebrahim. 1998. "Illness in the Context of Older Age: The Case of Stroke." *Sociology of Health & Illness* 20(4): 489–506.

Quittner, Alexandra L., David H. Barker, Ivette Cruz, Carolyn Snell, Mary E. Grimley, Melissa Botteri, and CDaCI Investigative Team. 2010. "Parenting Stress among Parents of Deaf and Hearing Children: Associations with Language Delays and Behavior Problems." *Parenting: Science and Practice* 10 (2): 136–155.

Ramsey, Claire, and José Antonio Noriega. 2001. "'*Niños Milagrizados*': Language Attitudes, Deaf Education, and Miracle Cures in Mexico." *Sign Language Studies* 1(3): 254–80.

Reynolds Whyte, Susan, and Benedicte Ingstad. 2007. "Introduction: Disability Connections." In *Disability in Local and Global Worlds,* ed. Benedicte Ingstad and Susan Reynolds Whyte, 1–29. Berkeley, CA: University of California Press.

Rosen, R. S. 2003. "Jargons for Deafness as Institutional Constructions of the Deaf Body." *Disability Society* 18(7): 921.

Salazar, N. 2012. "Tourism Imaginaries: A Conceptual Approach." *Annals of Tourism Research* 39(2): 863–82.

Skelton, Tracey, and Gill Valentine. 2003. "'It Feels Like Being Deaf is Normal': An Exploration into the Complexities of Defining D/Deafness and Young D/Deaf People's Identities." *Canadian Geographer* 47(4): 451.

Smith, Timothy B., Matthew N. I. Oliver, and Mark S. Innocenti. 2001. "Parenting Stress in Families of Children with Disabilities." *American Journal of Orthopsychiatry* 71 (2): 257.

Sökefeld, Martin. 1999. "Debating Self, Identity, and Culture in Anthropology." *Current Anthropology* 40(4): 417–448.

Todd, S., and S. Jones. 2005. "Looking at the Future and Seeing the Past: The Challenge of the Middle Years of Parenting a Child with Intellectual Disabilities." *Journal of Intellectual Disability Research* 49(6): 389–404.

Valentine, Gill. 2007. "Theorizing and Researching Intersectionality: A Challenge for Feminist Geography." *The Professional Geographer* 59(1): 10–21.

Van Deusen-Phillips, Sarah, Susan Goldin-Meadow, and Peggy J. Miller. 2001. "Enacting Stories, Seeing Worlds: Similarities and Differences in the Cross- Cultural Narrative Development of Linguistically Isolated Deaf Children." *Human Development* 44: 311-336.

Vindrola-Padros, C., and E. Brage. 2017. "What Is Not, But Might Be: The Disnarrated in Parents' Stories of Their Child's Cancer Treatment." *Social Science & Medicine* 193: 16–22.

White, N. R., and P. B. White. 2004. "Travel as Transition: Identity and Place." *Annals of Tourism Research* 31(1): 200–18.

Williams, G. 1984. "The Genesis of Chronic Illness: Narrative Re-construction." *Sociology of Health and Illness* 6(2): 175–200.

Wilson, S. 2007. "'When You Have Children, You're Obliged to Live': Motherhood, Chronic Illness and Biographical Disruption." *Sociology of Health & Illness* 29(4): 610–26.

Woodward, Kathryn. 1997. *Identity and Difference*. London: Sage in association with the Open University.

Young, B., M. Dixon-Woods, M. Findlay, and D. Heney. 2002. "Parenting in a Crisis: Conceptualising Mothers of Children with Cancer." *Social Science & Medicine* 55(10): 1835–47.

Zlatev, J. 2007. "Language, Embodiment and Mimesis." In *Body, Language and Mind: Vol 1. Embodiment,* ed. T. Ziemke, J. Zlatev, and R. Frank, 297–338. Berlin: Mouton de Gruyter.

CHAPTER
5

Egg Donor
Social Mobility and Expansion of Czech Reproductive Medicine

Amy Speier

I am sitting in a Prague fertility clinic located in a functionalist gray concrete hospital building on the outskirts of the Czech Republic's capital. The head nurse called me the previous week to inform me when Czech egg donors would be at the clinic to pick up their medications for their cycles.[1] I sit in a sterile, unoccupied nurse's office across the hall from the main nurse's office. Once the egg donors are finished with their checkups, the nurse sends them to me. As I sit across a desk from each egg donor, I haltingly explain my research project as I trip over Czech words with several consonants strung together. With the women who express interest in participating, I inquire about how they found out about egg donation, their motivations, and their reactions to the process. We touch on issues of anonymous egg donation, the pros and cons of whether their intended recipients are Czech or foreign patients, and their experiences with the clinics. After speaking with over thirty Czech egg donors, I come to realize that egg donation is a new form of mobile, part-time employment for young Czech women within a rapidly expanding market of Czech reproductive medicine.

In this chapter, I trace the explosion of the reproductive travel industry of the Czech Republic. Essentially, the Czech Republic's reproductive medical field has shifted from a domestic market to an international one, expanding to reach intended parents from all over the world. Intended parents are couples who usually suffer from infertility and resort to third-party assistant reproductive technologies in order to create a pregnancy, in this case relying on an egg and/or sperm donor. This newer stage of development reveals the fast-growing trend of medical tourism in countries like the Czech Republic. As a result of this expanding industry, Czech clinics have shifted their strategies for recruitment of egg donors.

Given the Czech Republic's relatively small population of 10.5 million, fertility clinics rely on new forms of recruitment of Czech egg donors. This chapter focuses on the "cultural mobilities" (Salazar 2010) of Czech egg donors. Underscoring the fact that there is a relationship between "culturally rooted imaginaries of mobility and real physical movements" (Salazar 2010, 53), I attempt to trace the cultural meanings that infuse Czech donor mobility. Furthermore, I frame mobility as a form of social practice (Vindrola-Padros and Johnson 2015: 1). While Vindrola-Padros and Johnson employ the term "micro-mobility" to capture children's individual health-seeking practice, in the case of cross-border reproductive care, egg donors are not seeking health services. Nevertheless, the authors insist that we must consider both the desire to move and the capacity to move as "tools" that Czech egg donors utilize. Throughout this chapter, I reveal how regional, social, economic, and imagined movements occur on various scales that are at times iterative and at other times cyclical. Young, childless Czech women and women on maternity leave are accessing new, flexible types of financial gain via egg donation that in turn enable even more social and cultural mobility. This chapter contextualizes the social mobility of Czech egg donors in a "particular political, economic, historical, and cultural context" (Vindrola-Padros and Johnson 2015: 3).

Methods

Other scholars have written about the difficulty of tracking international intended parents who are traveling for reproductive technologies (Inhorn 2004; Whittaker and Speier 2010). Understandably, infertility is a very private form of suffering, and many clinics aim to protect their patients. Trying to track egg donors in anonymous markets proved to be difficult as well. As with the case of couples traveling abroad for care, anthropologists must rely on third parties, such as agencies, clinics, doctors or brokers, to make contact with intended parents as well as with egg donors. I relied on a man who has close connections within the Czech reproductive medical world. He kindly introduced me to several clinics located in Prague, since I had previously worked only in Moravia.

During the summers of 2014 and 2015, I spent several months working with three fertility clinics in Prague. I conducted thirty-two semistructured interviews with Czech egg donors. In one clinic, where the squiggly lights hanging above the receptionist vaguely intimated sperm, I recruited former donors to come back to the clinic over the course of several days to speak with me in a large conference room. I sat in front of a world map entitled "Naše Děti ve Světě [Our children in the world]." Pushpins, each with a very small image of a stick figure baby on its head, were stuck in the countries of clients' geographic origins. Another clinic gave me the contact information of former egg donors, whom I contacted and met in public spaces. At the clinic introduced at the beginning of this chapter, which I call Orange, the nurse informed me when they expected egg donors to come to pick up their medications. After their appointments, I would tell them about my research project and ask if they wanted to be interviewed. In each instance, I went over the Czech informed consent form with each woman and sought her signature before we recorded our semistructured interviews. I have used pseudonyms for all donors and clinics. In addition to the thirty-two interviews I conducted with Czech egg donors, I also became a member of a closed Facebook group for 3,600 Czech egg donors, and I have tracked the posts on this page over the course of six months.

Early on in my interviews, I quickly learned that Czech egg donors are a mobile population traveling from all over the country to donate in clinics in Prague. Thus, I faced the challenges that other scholars studying mobile populations have described. Like other anthropologists engaged in researching mobile populations, I had to alter traditional ethnographic methodologies. I conducted participant observation at the clinic, which I consider to resemble "sites of passage, transfer points, where populations and things are temporarily contained and arranged within stations, waiting rooms and baggage systems" (Salazar, Elliot, and Norum 2017: 9). The clinic was literally a site of transfer for gametes (eggs) from Czech women, most often moved internationally to intended parents from all over the world.

Neoliberal Expansion of the Czech Reproductive Medical Market

The first "test-tube baby" born in the Soviet bloc of eastern Europe was born in 1982 in Czechoslovakia. Reproductive medicine has been a growing field in the Czech Republic since the 1990s. After the fall of the Berlin Wall in 1989, the Czech Republic witnessed the privatization of many fertility clinics. By the end of the twentieth century, four thousand of all births in the Czech Republic were in vitro fertilization (IVF) births. It is estimated that 15 percent of Czech couples suffer infertility (Slepičková and Fučík

2009), and 3.5 percent of Czech babies are born via assisted reproduction (Kocourkova, Burcin, and Kucera 2014).[2] Europe has witnessed a general decline in birthrates alongside an aging population. As a result, the Czech government funds up to four cycles of IVF for married Czech women under the age of thirty, and it has recently been considering funding treatment for single women as well.

Over the past decade, Czech reproductive medicine has moved well past simply meeting domestic demand for assisted reproductive technologies. Given its central European location as well as its relatively lower price structure, it has become a European hub for international "reproductive tourists."[3] Typically, destination sites of fertility travel can offer medical infrastructure and expertise, certain regulatory frameworks, and lower wage structures, which allow reproductive technologies to be performed at competitive, lower costs. In addition to a sense of cultural familiarity, patients are often seeking services such as sex selection, surrogacy, and commercial ova donation.

There are well-known "hubs" of reproductive tourism; however, many of these hubs have just recently shut down to international patients. India was well known for its surrogacy market, offering some of the most affordable cycles at $20,000 (in comparison to $100,000 in the United States). On average, five thousand babies were born annually in India within the commercial surrogacy market. However, in November 2015, the government banned the service for foreign couples, responding to various critics who thought the market exploited poor Indian women. Earlier the same year, Thailand banned surrogacy for international couples after the media released two very controversial stories related to the commercial industry (Marks 2015).

The largest hub of reproductive travel for those seeking IVF using egg donation and/or surrogacy is the highly unregulated "baby business" of the United States (Spar 2006). The North American reproductive medical field is a multimillion-dollar industry. Despite readily available technologies, the exorbitant price of treatment—roughly $100,000 for surrogacy and $30,000 or more for IVF with egg donation—means that only a small percentage of intended parents can afford to travel to the United States for treatment. Even though nearly all assisted reproductive technologies are readily available in the United States, even lower- and middle-class Americans must travel outside of the country for treatment. The Czech Republic becomes a good destination for everyone shut out of the US market.

Czech clinics market themselves to patients seeking ova donation. Czech clinical websites advertise in English, German, French, Italian, and Russian, promising a ready availability of student egg donors with only a three-month waiting period. The Czech reproductive medical field profits from its lower price structure and liberal legislation stipulating that sperm and egg donation must be voluntary and anonymous. Donors cannot be paid for their eggs, but are offered attractive "compensatory payments" of approximately 20,000 Czech crowns ($840) for the discomfort involved in ovarian stimulation and oocyte retrieval.[4] The average monthly income in the Czech Republic is 28,000 Czech crowns.

The globalization of reproductive biotechnologies has created even newer tastes and desires, inciting desire for the bodies of "others" (though their difference is suppressed) (Cohen 2002). The phenomenon of cross-border reproductive care reflects a globally "stratified reproduction" that entails "the power relations by which some categories of people are empowered to nurture and reproduce, while others are disempowered" (Ginsburg and Rapp 1995: 3). Czech egg donors are desirable genetic producers because they are of European descent. The fact that Czech egg donors receive only a fraction of what North American egg donors do reveals inequalities embedded in the marketing of bioavailability, or the trade in women's eggs (Heng 2006, 2007). There is a class structure in the reproductive industry in which individuals are ranked and considered appropriate for different reproductive tasks (Heng 2006, 2007; Tober 2002: 157). Compounding this fact is the idea that often "one woman's possession of reproductive choice may actually depend on or deepen another woman's reproductive vulnerability" (Solinger 2001: 7). In other words, the regional and global circulation of reproductive gametes (ova, sperm) brings stratification into sharp relief. "Even the reproductive body parts—the ova, sperm and embryos—are stratified and marketed according to their place of origin, the characteristics of their donors, and gender" (Whittaker and Speier 2010: 365). Czech egg donors are highlighted as white, European, and beautiful. This chapter considers the ways that stratified reproduction enables the global mobility of American, European, and Australian intended parents. In turn, reproductive travel engenders new kinds of economic, cultural, and geographic mobility for Czech egg donors, who supply this global market with their genetic material.

Reproductive travel has grown as one of the main forms of medical tourism because of the high cost of infertility treatment in the United States (Spar 2006; Thompson 2005), the unavailability of gamete donors due to regulations in places like Germany (Bergmann 2011), and strict regulatory laws like those in Italy (Zanini 2011). Those intended parents at the point in their fertility journey where they are considering IVF using an egg donor may suddenly find themselves barred from pursuing further treatment at home. Many couples on the market for an egg donor are from Australia, Europe, and North America. Given the "patchwork of widely diverging national laws" related to assisted reproductive technologies, a global industry has emerged that consists of a multitude of "varied" routes (Klotz and Knecht 2012: 284). A recent journal issue on cross-border reproductive care includes twenty-two nations and five continents (Gürtin and Inhorn 2011). It is impossible to know the exact numbers of patients traveling for reproductive care, nor how many people are traveling from particular locations (Nygren et al. 2010).

In 2012, it was said that 24,000 to 30,000 cycles of IVF were being performed in Europe each year (Inhorn and Patrizio 2012). The Czech Republic is emerging as one of the top European destinations for reproductive travel, because it offers anonymous egg donation; in contrast, other countries may stipulate that a child born of egg donation will have access to the donor's identity at age eighteen. Spain is the largest and oldest provider of reproductive medicine to foreign patients in Europe, and the Czech industry largely mimics the Spanish model. "Western civilization depends on IVF," a Czech doctor I interviewed proudly proclaimed. In response to this beckoning call, the Czech Republic has witnessed an explosion of fertility clinics all over the country. Over the past ten years, the number of fertility clinics has grown from twenty-five to forty-three (in a nation of ten million), which attests to the high level of demand for assisted reproductive technologies (ARTs) not only at home but also from many other countries. In 2007, 17,000 cycles of IVF were completed in the Czech Republic, while in 2013, there were 27,000—40 percent of which were for foreign couples (CTK 2016b). Given the cited numbers of cycles in Europe generally speaking, the Czech Republic's numbers are staggering. Czech clinics, most of them privately funded, are scattered across the nation. Some are nestled in border towns or situated in urban centers, while others appear in university towns with easy access to student donors ("Kde vám pomuzou" 2016).

Between 2010 and 2012, Czech clinics advertised heavily for egg donors—on trams, in school bulletins, and on local radio shows. It seems, however, that their social media marketing has morphed into a much larger phenomenon of snowball recruitment, whereby previous egg donors are telling other women about it and about the potential money they can make.[5] The overwhelming majority of my informants, 72 percent, knew someone who had donated, or they knew someone who worked at a fertility clinic. My previous work considers the importance of North American fertility tourist testimonials as essential for continuing the global fertility route to Czech fertility clinics (Speier 2016). North American women suffering from infertility actively use social media to meet others facing similar struggles, to seek information on treatment options, and as a site of advocacy for patient activism (Speier 2016). Thus, I was dumbstruck when I was sitting with my second informant, Barbora, at the main train station in a small restaurant near the shop where she worked. During her lunch break, she told me about a Facebook page for Czech egg donors. While I was well aware of the role the Internet played for patients looking to travel abroad for care, I had not anticipated this parallel world where egg donors would be seeking out similar types of support and information. Like couples seeking IVF abroad, Czech egg donors considering donation can choose from a total of forty-three Czech clinics.

Donors inform their decisions through recommendations from previous egg donors, whether in a closed Facebook group or from a close friend. In fact, 28 percent of my informants had learned about the possibility of egg donation online. These recommendations are akin to patient testimonials. I have talked about the "intimate labor" (Boris and Parreñas 2010) that is enacted by Czech clinics and coordinators for foreign patients, and how that "care" is central to what foreign patients are seeking. Intimate labor is a lens through which to examine the ways that global companies like fertility clinics must be nurturing to clients while earning a profit. At the same time, Czech egg donors want to know that they, too, will be cared for. Thus, the "intimate labor" enacted by Czech clinicians extends to both donors and clients. Czech clinics are relying heavily upon egg donor testimonials in order to garner further bio-sourcing material for their profits. The active use of the Internet by clinics, patients, and donors adds another dimension to this testimonial and the phenomena described here. Also, the fact that women are traveling between different clinics garners them flexible employment and identities.

Czech Egg Donors

The ages of the thirty-two Czech donor-participants ranged from eighteen to thirty-three. Clinics usually prefer that donors be at least nineteen years of age, and thirty-three is the cutoff. Nearly half of my informants (47 percent) were single, 9 percent were divorced, nearly 20 percent lived with a partner, and 16 percent were married.

During the spring of 2016, I began a project working with an egg donor search company in North America. I conducted two weeks of participant observation at its northern California office, participating in the Monday morning and Thursday afternoon meetings and also conducting semistructured interviews with the nine employees and two owners of the company. Based on my observations and conversations, I was amazed by the desire most intended parents had for a "smart" donor. The North American standards for "smart" are interpreted from SAT scores or GPA scores, as well as the type of educational institution one attends, with a preference for Ivy League universities. Somewhat similarly, Czech clinic advertisements assure intended parents that their donors are largely university students. Based on my sample, however, this may be false advertising. Only two of my informants had completed university and three were current university students. The Czech Republic does have a different educational system, whereby primary school is until age fifteen, at which point students may enter secondary high school or a vocational school, some with exit exams and some without. The majority of my informants, 53 percent, had completed vocational or high school, while two had completed only primary school.

In addition, many egg donors are mothers. Clinics tend to prefer donors who are already mothers, since it means they are "proven" donors.[6] While I spoke with Barbora at the train station, she admitted she was not sure if she would have children since she had not yet found anyone to have them with. Despite her childlessness, she said, "It is also better when a woman already has a child because then it is tested that her eggs are working good [*sic*]." However, half of my informants were childless, with most of them declaring that they did want children in the future; only 12 percent claimed, like Barbora, that they were uncertain. Of those who had children, half were single mothers. In addition, nearly a quarter of my informants were on maternity leave. As a North American, I was stunned by the vast difference between maternity leave policies of the Czech Republic and those of North America. Whereas most women in the United States may have up to six weeks of unpaid leave from work, Czech women can receive up to three years of maternity leave, though they must take a fraction of their salary in the second and third years.

There seems to be no Czech national registry that is used to limit the number of times a woman can donate her eggs. Thus, I met donors who were donating for the first time as well as donors who were donating for the fifth time. Some clinics only allow a Czech woman to donate three times, yet there are no regulatory frameworks to enforce this rule. Furthermore, there are no regulatory practices among clinics to ensure that a woman is not donating at clinic A, B, and C. Indeed, I witnessed many women who circulated all over the country, traveling from clinic to clinic donating—their geographic mobility sometimes repetitive and sometimes circuitous and based on others' recommendations of "care" offered by nurses and clinics.

I asked my interviewees if they knew of any particular limit in terms of egg donors. Some replied that they thought women could donate only until they were thirty-three, or only once every three to four months, which indicated to me that women tend to donate more than one time. Of my respondents, 34 percent were first-time egg donors, although many planned to do it again in the future, and 34 percent had donated twice, while the rest had donated upward of three times. For this reason, I argue that we must consider egg donation a form of part-time employment. What is also interesting to note is that for those fifteen participants who thought there may be a limit (e.g., a woman should donate only three or six times), they usually offered a caveat related to the fact that it is an "individual choice" or it depends on the woman's "health." For example, Blanka, a twenty-one-year-old single woman without children, believed a woman should only donate twice if she has not had children, but then immediately added, "Each person should decide how many times." This individualistic attitude regarding the risks associated with egg donation reflects a more pervasive ideology about individual responsibility for one's health.[7] In previous work, I have shown how patients traveling abroad for healthcare assume this personal responsibility (Speier 2016), and I see it also occurring in conversations with egg donors. Their notions reflect neoliberal ideas of the market, recalling the ways that Czech factory workers and managers spoke of their employment in a newly "free market" (Weiner 2007).

Economic Mobility

Various scholars have written about the motivations for egg donors, debating how gamete donation may be closely aligned with blood donation, or whether it must be considered a gift economy or a market transaction. I decided to ask my informants what compelled them to donate. Very often, they would mention someone they knew—a friend, a family member, or a colleague—who had had a hard time getting pregnant, and so they wanted to help. They may have wanted to help a particular person, yet then came to find out that donation in the Czech Republic is anonymous and they could not help anyone they know.

While most said that they wanted to help, they also frankly admitted that the money was nice as well. Only two women simply said they donated for the money. Most often, women said it was a combination of both. One Czech egg donor responded, "I guess that there are two reasons: one is that you help someone else—those who can't get pregnant naturally; and the money also always helps. I'd be lying if I said it is not true." Very similarly, the next woman I met said, "I will be honest: the money comes first. And when you can help someone in that way, then you say 'why not?'" There may be some level of socialization of the egg donors by the clinics in terms of encouraging them to donate because they will "help" someone, somewhat similar to the socialization of surrogates in North America. In her recent ethnography, Jacobson (2016) writes about the reluctance of surrogates to refer to their pregnancies as a form of employment, preferring to speak in terms of a "calling."

Conversations concerning this issue of monetary compensation appear frequently on the closed Facebook page. I have only witnessed one woman who posted that she was glowing for having given someone a chance at happiness. Other women quickly chimed in saying that this group simply would not exist if it were not for the compensation. I noted how other women replied that their first donation was for altruistic reasons, yet the subsequent donations were for money. Given the fact that donation earns Czech women nearly one month's salary, many are inclined to donate several times for the flexible spending it affords.

During my first summer of research, in 2010, when I began another project focusing on North Americans traveling to the Czech Republic for IVF, I met with an IVF coordinator at a small Moravian clinic. Lenka, the wife of a doctor at the clinic, surmised that Czech women donate their eggs for the money. There was no squeamishness in saying that this was their motivation, and she explained that Czech donors clearly distinguish between an egg and a child. Lenka bluntly said to me, "I never met donor who would do that from my point of view from just altruistic reasons. It is all about money, and they are not as sensitive as I should say they should be. . . . [T]hey just ask when they get the money. That's why I don't think that that they really realize what they are doing." Another scholar, who compares egg and sperm donation in a North American context, has also written about this issue of motivation. She found that while critics will denounce financial motivations of egg donors, students tend to have a bit more leeway if they are financially motivated, since the money is supposedly going toward their education (Almeling 2006: 153). In the global reproductive medical industry, there is a general resistance to acknowledging the financial transactions taking place, as people tend to want to paint a more altruistic picture of egg donation. Thus, students are not judged as harshly as a woman who may not be working, because the money is deemed to be going toward a valuable end. In fact, some Czech egg donors are indeed looking for ways to pay for their education.

The clinic in Zlín has five hundred women who are potential egg donors, which, according to Lenka, is an overflow and more than they need. The clinical doctors categorize donors into large groups based on genetic history, health, looks, and level of education. Lenka explains, "A is perfect, pass, more than average, B is average, and C is not very good . . . and because we have so many donors, we really do not have a need. They are in the database. We have some Cs, but I do not have a need to call her because I still have enough As and Bs." Women often call the clinic to inquire about the possibility of donating their eggs. As in the case of the United States, there is an "oversupply of women willing to be egg donors . . . far outstripping recipient demand. Despite this abundance, egg donor fees hold steady and are often calibrated by staff perceptions of a woman's characteristics and a recipient's wealth" (Almeling 2007: 336).

Americans often wonder aloud about the stark price difference of IVF in the Czech Republic compared to the United States, but do not focus on the fact that Czech egg donors are paid significantly less than American donors. Waldby and Mitchell (2006: 8), among others, have shown how "a transfer of tissues from one person to another follows the trajectories of power and wealth, as the poor sell their body parts to those with more wealth." These authors complicate the dichotomy of framing human tissue donation in terms of either a gift or commodity system. Such a dichotomy fails to take into account "the political economy of the modern world of globalized biotechnology" (Waldby and Mitchell 2006: 9). In fact, "gift and commodity systems interpenetrate each other in increasingly complex ways" (p. 25). Like human tissue, egg donation is both gift and commodity exchange, signaling an overlap as with the intimate labor provided by suppliers of this global reproductive travel industry.

As I strolled the cobblestone sidewalks of Prague last summer with a close Czech friend the night before I was to return home, she said there are very few part-time jobs available to women who have small children. In fact, only 6 percent of the work in the Czech Republic is part-time (CTK 2016a), which is one of the lowest shares in the European Union, which averages 30 percent of work as part-time. Even further, gaps in workforce participation between men and women are significant; there is an 18.7 percent difference in pay rate between men and women (Sprincova and Adamusova 2010); and the unemployment rate for women is 8 percent, whereas for men it is 5.9 percent (Roland Berger Strategy Consultants 2013). More often than not, those women working part-time are mothers of young children, who need to combine care of the family and children and/or older family members with some sort of employment. Those who are working part-time would prefer full-time employment (CTK 2016a). I argue that we must consider egg donation as a recent and increasingly appealing option for young mothers and women who cannot necessarily find part-time employment. Given the general dearth of part-time employment opportunities for Czechs, as well as clinical preferences for egg donors who are young mothers, and the speed by which word of mouth has spread among women who promote egg donation as a way to quickly earn money, egg donation can be understood as an employment opportunity. Moreover, it is a flexible and mobile form of labor.

Reproductive technologies are traversing the globe at rapid speeds, and patients are crossing international borders to seek treatment that may not be available to them at home. An unexpected finding of this research was the extent of travel in which Czech egg donors are engaged during their donation cycles. Although my research took place at three different Prague fertility clinics, women were traveling from all over the Czech Republic, some taking 5.5-hour-long train rides from the north, or 3-hour car rides from Western Bohemia with friends who were also donating. Despite the fact that there are often clinics closer to their homes near the national borders, women understand Prague to be the highest-paying city and they are willing to travel. We see how technologies and people—both patients and donors—are mobile in different ways within the reproductive healthcare system in the Czech Republic. This mobility may also be spurred on by a cultural imagination of Prague as a metropolitan hub.

As the global market for reproductive travel expands, and the Czech market grows steadily to treat foreign couples seeking egg donation, a new category of young women who are not yet mothers is entering a highly mobile employment domain. Alena was a twenty-four-year-old university student who did not have children. She planned to go on holiday with the money she made from her second egg donation. She said, "I don't really know yet what kind of a career I would like to have. I still have time. Right now I would like to go for a vacation and when I return, I will need to decide whether to quit my job and get a new one. . . . I live alone. Because I have a job I got used to making some money, so I don't lead a typical student life—I like to buy nice things—nice handbags, shoes . . . so that's about it." The expanding industry of reproductive travel seems to have incited a new kind of economic and geographic mobility for young Czech women—both for mothers on maternity leave without other options for employment and for young women who are earning cash for leisure. Thus, we witness at least two forms of mobility that intersect for donors who are seeking cash to travel. There is the geographic mobility that enables college students to leave home and live in a new, perhaps more metropolitan city. Other types of discretionary income are also offered by the compensation for donating one's eggs. In other words, not only do women gain employment, but they also find real ways to actualize their desires for social or geographic mobility.

The Health and Care of Egg Donors

While egg donors are not seeking any particular treatment when visiting a clinic, and the long-term effects of the medications on their bodies remains unknown, they still gain knowledge about their own health status based on notions of genetics and hereditary diseases. Helena, twenty-three, said, "I didn't come here for the money. I wanted to help someone and find out how I am doing with those tests." If we want to follow up on the question of altruism, to put it very starkly, Helena was seeking genetic information that she desired and imagined useful for her own sense of well-being. She had learned about egg donation on Facebook and was interested in learning from the genetic tests, since her grandmother had gradually been paralyzed and her grandfather was shortsighted. It seems as if the global travel of intended parents wanting to create particular kinds of families through IVF using egg donation is enabling a new form of genealogical knowledge for Czech egg donors (Nash 2003). Also, for Helena, Ostrava was closer but she would rather travel to Prague, where she had friends. Thus, egg donors are choosing clinics based on favorable locations and compensation. Egg donor regional mobility reflects imaginations of Prague or other cities that lure donors there for cultural and historical reasons.

Some informants that I spoke with thought clinics were looking for someone with "regular" looks, which proved to be another difference I have noted in comparison to the American "baby business" (Spar 2006). Employees of search agencies in the United States often talked about how intended parents wanted smart and "good looking" donors. If Czech donors believe that the clinics either want features that "match" those of an intended parent or are simply looking for someone "regular" with no "oddities," then the process of egg donation may be reaffirming their sense of normality. By learning that they are "regular," they also feel accepted; as Barbora said, "They picked me, I guess they liked me." Donors were essentially getting confirmation of their good health and regularity and feedback on their desirability through indirect commentary on their physical looks. These notions of self, health, and acceptance are tools that can enable donors to envision potential future social mobility—a social mobility that is engendered by a culturally rooted imaginary fueled by the demand for their genetic material.

Conclusion

The reproductive medical industry of the Czech Republic has exploded during the past decade. The Czech Republic is a favorite destination of intended parents from all over Europe, North America, and Australia. Most couples traveling to the Czech Republic for fertility treatment are seeking IVF using egg donors. This chapter provided a glimpse into a sample of young Czech women who are supplying this global industry of human reproductive material. Czech mothers are banking on their bioavailability to take care of their families and young children while they are on maternity leave; single women take advantage of this option to be able to take small holidays and have "nice things." I have employed the term "cultural mobility" (Salazar

2010) in this chapter to capture the varying levels of geographic, social, and economic mobility of egg donors that the global reproductive travel market engenders for young women. This mobility is infused with cultural meaning (Salazar 2010: 55). As in Salazar's (2010: 57) study of cultural mobility in Tanzania, Czech egg donors' migratory patterns to Prague tend to reflect a circular form of mobility attached to the capital center of the country.

Given the paucity of part-time employment opportunities as well as the gendered nature of part-time work, for some women egg donation has proven to be a viable option for flexible work. Young women are traversing the Czech Republic, traveling to various clinics to donate several times in order to earn as much as the average monthly income for each cycle. Their regional, cyclical institutional movement is directly tied to their financial and social mobility. Czech egg donors, like intended parents, are turning to the Internet to seek information as well as support for their new ventures into egg donation as a form of employment. We may consider their participation in these online forums as a response to their new flexible labor. Their geographic mobility is a response to the mobile nature of the cross-border reproductive care industry. The overlapping and iterative geographic, financial, and social mobility of Czech egg donors is spurred on by their own culturally rooted imaginaries of travel and their identities as young working women in a flexible global economy.

Amy Speier, PhD, is a medical anthropologist specializing in reproductive health, globalization, and medical tourism, and the author of *Fertility Holidays: IVF Tourism and the Reproduction of Whiteness* (New York University Press, 2016). In the book, she examines the multiple motivations that compel infertile couples to travel halfway across the globe in their quest for parenthood. She conducted a multiyear, multisited ethnographic research project tracing North American fertility travels to the Czech Republic, and she is now looking at tracing global journeys to North America in search of fertility treatments.

NOTES

1. An IVF "cycle" includes shutting down a woman's natural cycle of egg production in the ovaries, stimulating the ovaries to produce more than one egg, retrieving the egg from the woman's ovaries, collecting the man's sperm, fertilizing the eggs with the sperm in a lab, incubating the fertilized eggs for up to five days (blastocyst), and transferring one or two of the healthiest embryos into a woman's uterus.
2. For a sense of comparison, slightly more than 1.5 percent of all births in the United States are born via ARTs. One reason for the higher percentage in the Czech Repub-

lic is that most Czech women using IVF are younger than thirty-five, which means there is a higher success rate of live births.

3. Scholars have debated the terminology of fertility tourism, referring to it as "reproductive tourism," "procreative tourism," or "cross-border reproductive care" (Gürtin and Inhorn 2011; Whittaker and Speier 2010).
4. For comparison, women in North American can earn anywhere from $5,000 to $8,000 per cycle, yet there is no limit.
5. Based on preliminary research in North America, this method of recruitment has also proven useful for egg donor agencies.
6. In the Ukraine, for example, only mothers are accepted as egg donors.
7. Possible risks associated with egg donation result from fertility drugs, which may cause bloating, headache, mood shifts, and ovarian hyperstimulation syndrome (OHSS), which can (rarely) lead to death.

REFERENCES

Almeling, R. 2006. "'Why Do You Want to Be a Donor?': Gender and the Production of Altruism in Egg and Sperm Donation." *New Genetics and Society* 25(2): 143–57.

———. 2007. "Selling Genes, Selling Gender: Egg Agencies, Sperm Banks, and the Medical Market in Genetic Materials." *American Sociological Review* 72(3): 319–40.

Bergmann, S. 2011. "Reproductive Agency and Projects: Germans Searching for Egg Donation in Spain and the Czech Republic." *Reproductive BioMedicine Online* 23(5): 600–8.

Boris, E., and R. S. Parreñas. 2010. "Introduction." In *Intimate Labors: Cultures, Technologies, and the Politics of Care,* ed. E. Boris and R.S. Parreñas, 1–12. Stanford, CA: Stanford University Press.

Cohen, L. 2002. "The Other Kidney: Biopolitics beyond Recognition." In *Commodifying Bodies,* ed. N. Scheper-Hughes and L. Wacquant, 9–30. London: SAGE.

CTK. 2016a. "One-Fifth of Czechs Working Part-Time Do So Involuntarily." *Prague Daily Monitor,* 7 March. Retrieved 2 August 2016 from http://www.praguemonitor.com/2016/03/07/one-fifth-czechs-working-part-time-do-so-involuntarily.

———. 2016b. "Asistovaná Reprodukce je v CR Dostupnejsí." *Ozdravotnictví,* 11 March. Retrieved 21 March 2016 from https://www.ozdravotnictvi.cz/zpravodajstvi/asistovana-reprodukce-je-v-cr-dostupnejsi/.

Ginsburg, F.D., and R. Rapp. 1995. "Introduction." *Conceiving the New World Order: The Global Politics of Reproduction,* ed. F. D. Ginsburg and R. Rapp, 1–18. Berkeley: University of California Press.

Gürtin, Z.B., and M.C. Inhorn, eds. 2011. "Symposium: Cross-Border Reproductive Care." Special issue, *Reproductive BioMedicine Online* 23(5).

Heng, B.C. 2006. "'Reproductive Tourism': Should Locally Registered Fertility Doctors Be Held Accountable for Channeling Patients to Foreign Medical Establishments?" *Human Reproduction* 21(3): 840–42.

———. 2007. "Regulatory Safeguards Needed for the Traveling Foreign Egg Donor." *Human Reproduction* 22(8): 2350–2.

Inhorn, M.C. 2004. "Privacy, Privatization, and the Politics of Patronage: Ethnographic Challenges to Penetrating the Secret World of Middle Eastern, Hospital-Based In Vitro Fertilization." *Social Science & Medicine* 59(10): 2095–108.

Inhorn, M.C., and P. Patrizio. 2012. "The Global Landscape of Cross-Border Reproductive Care: Twenty Key Findings for the New Millennium." *Current Opinion Obstetrics and Gynecology* 24(3): 158–63.

Jacobson, H. 2016. *Gestational Surrogacy and the Work of Making Babies.* New Brunswick, NJ: Rutgers University Press.

"Kde vám pomuzou." *Stop Neplodnosti.cz.* Retrieved 2 August 2016 from http://www.stopneplodnosti.cz/kde-vam-pomohou.

Klotz, M., and M. Knecht. 2012. "What Is Europeanization in the Field of Assisted Reproductive Technologies?" In *Reproductive Technologies as Global Form: Ethnographies of Knowledge, Practices, and Transnational Encounters,* ed. M. Knecht, M. Klotz, and S. Beck, 283–302. Frankfurt: Campus Verlag GmbH.

Kocourkova, J., B. Burcin, and T. Kucera. 2014. "Demographic relevancy of increased use of assisted reproduction in European countries." In *Reproductive Health,* 26 May. Retrieved 23 March 2018 from https://www.ncbi.nlm.nih.gov/pmc/articles/PMC4049397/.

Marks, K. 2015. "Baby Gammy: Australian Father Who Abandoned Down Syndrome Surrogate Child Now Tries to Access Funds Donated for His Care." *Independent,* 19 May. Retrieved 2 August 2016 from http://www.independent.co.uk/news/world/australasia/baby-gammy-australian-father-who-abandoned-down-syndrome-surrogate-child-now-tries-to-access-funds-10261916.html.

Nash, C. 2003. "'They're Family!': Cultural Geographies of Relatedness in Popular Genealogy." In *Uprootings/Regroundings: Questions of Home and Migration,* ed. S. Ahmed, C. Castañeda, and A. Fortie, 179–203. Oxford: Berg.

Nygren, K., D. Adamson, F. Zegers-Hochschild, J. de Mouzon, and International Committee Monitoring Assisted Reproductive Technologies. 2010. "Cross-Border Fertility Care—International Committee Monitoring Assisted Reproductive Technologies Global Survey: 2006 Data and Estimates." *Fertility and Sterility* 94(1): e4–e10.

Roland Berger Strategy Consultants. 2013. "The Current Situation of Equality in the Czech Republic - Country Profile." Retrieved 2 August 2016 from http://ec.europa.eu/justice/gender-equality/files/epo_campaign/country_profile_czech_republic_en.pdf.

Salazar, N.B. 2010. "Towards an Anthropology of Cultural Mobilities." *Crossings: Journal of Migration and Culture* 1(1): 53–68.

Salazar, N.B., A. Elliot, and R. Norum. 2017. "Studying Mobilities: Theoretical Notes and Methodological Inquiries." In *Methodologies of Mobility: Ethnography and Experiment,* ed. A. Elliot, R. Norum, and N. B. Salazar, 1–24. New York: Berghahn Books.

Slepičková, L., and P. Fučík. 2009. "The Social Context of Attitudes toward Various Infertility Strategies." *Czech Sociological Review* 45(2): 267–90.

Solinger, B. 2001. *Beggars and Choosers: How the Politics of Choice Shapes Adoption, Abortion, and Welfare in the United States.* New York: Hill and Wang.

Spar, D. 2006. *The Baby Business: How Money, Science, and Politics Drive the Commerce of Conception.* Boston, MA: Harvard Business School Press.

Speier, A. 2016. *Fertility Holidays: IVF Tourism and the Reproduction of Whiteness.* New York: New York University Press.

Sprincova, V., and M. Adamusova. 2010. *Gender Equality in the Czech Republic: Working Paper.* Friedrich Ebert Stiftung. Accessed 23 March 2018. https://aa.ecn.cz/img_upload/666f72756d35302d6669313030313139/czech-republic_report_final_1.pdf.

Thompson, C. 2005. *Making Parents: The Ontological Choreography of Reproductive Technologies.* Boston, MA: MIT Press.

Tober, D.M. 2002. "Semen as Gift, Semen as Goods: Reproductive Workers and the Market in Altruism." in *Commodifying Bodies,* ed. N. Scheper-Hughes and L. Wacquant, 137–160. London: SAGE.

Vindrola-Padros, C., and G.A. Johnson. 2015. "Children Seeking Health Care: International Perspectives on Children's Use of Mobility to Obtain Health Services." In *Movement, Mobilities, and Journeys: Geographies of Children and Young People,* ed. C. N. Laoire, A. White, and T. Skelton, 289–306. Singapore: Springer.

Waldby, C., and R. Mitchell. 2006. *Tissue Economies: Blood, Organs, and Cell Lines in Late Capitalism.* Durham, NC: Duke University Press.

Weiner, E. 2007. *Market Dreams: Gender, Class, and Capitalism in the Czech Republic.* Ann Arbor, MI: University of Michigan Press.

Whittaker, A., and A. Speier. 2010. "'Cycling Overseas': Care, Commodification, and Stratification in Cross-Border Reproductive Travel." *Medical Anthropology* 29(4): 363–83.

Zanini, G. 2011. "Abandoned by the State, Betrayed by the Church: Italian Experiences of Cross-Border Reproductive Care." *Reproductive BioMedicine Online* 23(5): 565–72.

CHAPTER
6

Governing Mobility of Health Workers across Borders
From Local to Global Policy Tools

Evgeniya Plotnikova

The latest medicine and the newest technologies may have little impact on human health if there are not systems with skilled personnel in place to deliver healthcare services (WHO 2006a). The size, distribution, and composition of the health workforce have a crucial impact on the overall quality of health service delivery. Today, one of the key problems many health systems in both developed and developing countries share is a deficit and a maldistribution of health workers.[1] The World Health Organization (WHO) reports (2016a) that in 2013, there was an estimated global deficit of 17.6 million health workers, including medical doctors, nurses, midwives, and other health cadres. What are the reasons for the increasing scarcity in health personnel around the world? In developing countries, factors include a high share of global burden of disease, chronic underinvestment in health workforce training, and a massive outflow of health workers who are attracted to developed countries through the lure of higher salaries, better living conditions, and promising career opportunities abroad (Kline 2003).

In 2006, the WHO estimated that fifty-seven countries experienced a critical shortage in their health workforce, claiming fewer than 23 health workers per 10,000 of the population (WHO 2006b). Most of these countries were in the regions of Southeast Asia and sub-Saharan Africa. In the latter, the density of physicians, for instance, per 1,000 population ranges from 0.023 in Liberia to 0.096 in Ghana (WHO 2016b). However, shortages in health personnel are not limited to developing countries. Developed countries also report scarcity in health workers—to an extent that is perhaps less alarming than in developing countries, but still visible in health service delivery. For example, it is estimated that by 2025, the United States, one of the leading countries receiving health workers from abroad, will face the need for an additional 500,000 nurses and 44,000 family physicians (Campbell et al. 2014). Furthermore, it is predicted that European Union (EU) countries will face a shortage of one million health workers by 2020 (European Commission 2012).

A complex interplay of factors explains the global nature of health worker scarcity around the globe. Factors include demographic and epidemiological changes, political priorities, economic conditions, technological innovations, and consumer expectations (Kline 2003). The health workforce shortage in the majority of developed countries is seen as a periodically emerging gap between labor supply and demand (Clark, Stewart, and Clark 2006). This gap is a result of an imperfect health labor market model, in which the relevant adjustments take a longer amount of time than in competitive labor markets (Zurn et al. 2004). In these conditions, the imbalance between supply and demand is likely to become static in the long term. As with most other markets, the labor market for health workers is characterized by market failures, but of unique importance is the extent of these market failures. The labor market for the health workforce is particularly vulnerable for a number of reasons. First, both labor supply and labor demand rely on the sociodemographic structure of the population in general and the health workforce in particular. For instance, in developed countries, demand for long-term healthcare increases with growth in the older population. At the same time, aging of the health workforce leads to high retirement rates and decreased labor supply (Baumann et al. 2004). Second, reproduction of human resources for health is a time-consuming and costly process. Labor supply is affected by a substantial time lag between education and practice. For instance, an average of at least three years is required to train a nurse and, depending on a specialty, ten to fifteen years to train a doctor (Robinson and Griffiths 2007). Therefore, it takes years to see the results of an investment in health workforce education. Moreover, the introduction of more training places as an individual measure would not necessarily solve the problem of labor shortage. The stability of the workforce also depends upon whether the health profession attracts young talent and whether experienced staff are motivated to stay in practice despite professional hazards associated with healthcare, such as heavy workloads, night shifts, and psychological pressures. Third, the health workforce shortage is often a result of political decisions inspired by the cost-containment policy in the health service. For instance, in the early 1990s the Conservative government in the UK considerably reduced the number of training places for nurses; by the end of the decade, the staffing shortages in Britain had already become apparent (Buchan and Edwards 2000). A similar policy pattern of cutting the intake of nursing students was followed by the UK coalition government in 2010, contributing to nursing shortages reported in 2014–15 (Royal College of Nursing 2015).

The growing pressures placed on the health sector, and on individual providers of health services, produce various forms of labor mobility. These include intrasector transitions from public to private healthcare institutions; intersector mobility when professionals leave healthcare-related jobs and move to other occupations; and, finally, geographical mobility to foreign countries. The last of these forms of labor mobility, geographical mobility to foreign countries, significantly accelerated in the three decades preceding the financial crisis in 2008. As reported by the Organisation for Economic Co-operation and Development (OECD), in 2010–11 foreign doctors and foreign nurses accounted for more than 20 percent and 14 percent, respectively, of health workers in OECD countries. However, during the economic recession, this share of foreign health workers decreased, falling to 17 percent and 6 percent for doctors and nurses, respectively, by 2012–14 (OECD 2010, 2016). Although the financial crisis of 2008 and the increased focus on domestic training of health workers in many developed countries both have stabilized and even slowed down the pace of labor mobility in a number of countries, the systematic reliance on foreign-trained health workers continues to raise concerns. The growth of cross-border mobility of health workers since the 2000s has led to the re-establishment of a long-standing debate, which began in the early 1970s, around the problem of "brain drain" (Martineau, Decker, and Bundred 2004). Many questions that were posed four decades ago require further attention today: How many health workers move across borders each year? What policies can adequately manage health worker migration, secure access to health service in source countries, and protect rights of migrant health professionals?

This chapter focuses on the challenges of managing the cross-border mobility of health workers. It problematizes mobility as the object of regulation by exploring existing policy tools at the global, national, and local levels. It addresses two questions: (1) What tensions are created by the cross-border mobility of health workers? (2) How are these tensions addressed (or not) by policy tools?

Contemporary Trends: The Rise of Cross-Border Nurse Mobility

In the late 1990s and the early 2000s, the cross-border mobility of health workers increased significantly and reached a critical point. For example, the number of work permits granted to overseas nurses and doctors in the UK alone during the period from 2001 to 2006 was 147,640 and 17,779, respectively (Buchan, Baldwin, and Munro 2008). This can be compared to the estimates of overall health worker migration in 1978: 14,000 nurses moving across national borders and 140,000 physicians practicing outside their own countries (Mejia 1978). These data indicate a significant intensification of migration flows of international health workers today, not only to the UK, but worldwide. Moreover, these data point to a shift in occupational mobility, with nurses becoming more active labor migrants (Martineau et al. 2004; Stewart, Clark, and Clark 2007).

A group of factors contributes to expanding overseas employment opportunities for both nurses and medical professionals, including improved transportation links and relatively reduced travel costs; an increasing number of recruitment agencies mediating cross-border mobility; the proliferation of access to the Internet as a source of knowledge about jobs and employers; negotiation of government-to-government agreements facilitating migration flows; and international recognition of qualifications (Buchan, Seccombe, and Hutt 2006). The general trend of nurse migration, which had increased gradually since the 1970s, rocketed in the late 1990s. In an effort to address the temporary shortages in health personnel, many developed countries were actively recruiting from developing countries. As policy analysts have argued, this recruitment drive deepened the chronic crisis in human resources in health across the globe, particularly in poor regions such as sub-Saharan Africa (Kline 2003; Bourgain, Pieretti, and Zou 2008). A cycle was thus created whereby the shortage of nurses in developed countries stimulated outflow of health workers from the developing world and, as a consequence, contributed to the critical situation in their health systems. This provoked many criticisms of unethical recruitment practices by developed countries and fueled dialogues on how to respond to the health workforce crisis at a global level and mitigate the negative effects of health worker migration in developing countries (Dovlo 2005; WHO 2006a).

International Health Worker Mobility as a Regulatory Challenge

Discussion of the effective regulation of the cross-border mobility of health workers has been present in the policy discourse since the "brain drain" problem was originally exposed in the early 1970s (Martineau et al. 2004).

At that time, the phenomenon was portrayed as a national regulatory problem of controlling the number of labor migrants by using restriction, retention, and changes in health worker education systems as the key tools (Gish and Godfrey 1979). This debate continues today; however, the regulatory problem has now reached a new, global level, which requires a joint response from the governments of developed and developing countries and nonstate actors at the global and local levels.

The contemporary dynamics of international mobility of health workers, for both doctors and nurses, are often referred to as a "carousel movement" and "brain circulation" (Blitz 2005; Ncayiyana 1999). This type of migration is described in an OECD report that illustrates mobility patterns of South African physicians (OECD 2004). In contrast to the original conceptualization of health worker movement as one-directional, the OECD suggests a complex and multilayer picture of migratory routes when, for example, Canadian doctors move to the United States to work and are then replaced by South African doctors from urban areas. Meanwhile, the South African government covers the shortage of physicians in rural areas by recruiting Cuban doctors. Likewise, the United Kingdom, which loses health workers to North America, recruits from other European countries such as Germany, Poland, and Spain. At the same time, Germany receives doctors from central and eastern European countries, such as the Czech Republic (OECD 2004). A similar picture could be drawn to illustrate migration flows of nurse professionals. While many British nurses choose to work in Australia, the United States, and New Zealand, back home they are being replaced with recruits from the Philippines who receive nurse training in their home country as a response to strong migratory aspirations. The global demand for nurses also encourages Filipino physicians to retrain as nurses to advance their job opportunities abroad (Lorenzo et al. 2007). Often the migration journey of Filipino nurses starts in one of the Middle East countries such as Saudi Arabia or United Arab Emirates, where they improve their professional skills and save money for further travel to the UK; then, after practicing for couple of years, they move again to the United States—the final desired destination for many Filipino nurses (Kingma 2006).

To sum up, the literature tracking global mobility among health workers suggests that migratory patterns and final destinations are dependent upon multiple factors and in constant flux. The two examples above not only illustrate contemporary migratory routes of South African doctors and Filipino nurses, but also provide a snapshot of a more general trend in health personnel migration around the globe. The latter includes many stops in the migratory route between—and within—developed and developing countries, where one country often becomes a stepping stone for a move to another state. The complex and multilevel character of contemporary migration is only one of the challenges in the regulation of health worker mobility. A number of other factors contribute to and complicate the problem of effective governance in cross-border movement of health personnel: dramatic increases in flows of labor migration and the proliferation of private recruitment networks across geographical borders.

To further demonstrate why and how the governance of international health worker migration becomes a regulatory problem, this chapter employs the language of human rights (UN General Assembly 1948). On the one hand, it introduces the state's obligation to respect, protect, and fulfill the individual's right to health.[2] In particular, this analysis refers to the state's obligation to ensure that sufficient numbers of doctors and other health professionals are available in a country (OHCHR 2008). At the same time, it refers to the rights of migrant health workers to freedom of movement (the right to migrate) and free choice of employment, including overseas. The reference to human rights in the discussion of causes and implications of international migration of health workers is not new (Mesquita and Gordon 2005). Relatively recent attempts date back to the late 1990s and early 2000s, when a number of meetings were organized at the international level to discuss the negative impacts of health worker migration and the effective regulation of it (Plotnikova 2011). The migration and recruitment of health workers was seen as a controversial process, causing a conflict between the right to health of patients in source countries and the right to freedom of movement of health workers. The right to health appeared in the rhetoric of various stakeholders at national and international levels. For instance, international organizations considered active international recruitment to be one of the key factors affecting the right to health of patients in developing countries (WHO Executive Board 2004). The implementation of the right to health was reinforced by General Comment 14 of the International Covenant on Economic, Social and Cultural Rights (ICESCR), which emphasizes that protection of the right to health is an obligation of national governments (UNCESCR 2000). According to the ICESCR, states should implement policies that lead to available and accessible healthcare for all and ensure that third parties conform to human rights standards. Governments in source countries actively used this interpretation of the right to health to accuse developed countries of "poaching" health workers (Stilwell 2009). Those making such accusations further demanded that active recruitment be stopped and that developed countries compensate the loss of valuable human resources either by direct financial transfers or through investment in the training of health workers in developing countries. Many of these demands were directed at the British government, whose public and private institutions actively recruited foreign doctors and nurses in the late 1990s and early 2000s (discussed further in the following section). At the same time, professional organizations and trade unions in source countries supported the right of health workers to leave their country of origin in search of better career opportunities. However, they also condemned the practices of employers in developed countries who were actively recruiting workers from developing countries. For instance, despite explicit government support for labor emigration, professional organizations and trade unions in the Philippines and India expressed criticisms of the recruitment of their health workers (Galvez-Tan 2005).

This controversy of arguments around international migration of health personnel exposed a long-standing opposition between the state and the health profession (Johnson 1995). On the one hand, claims to stop active recruitment as well as certain national policies, such as "bonding" (an obligation to practice after graduation in public institutions and/or rural areas), are adopted by the governments of source countries to protect the sustainability of national health systems and to ensure that an appropriate number of health workers are retained in the country. On the other hand, these policies affect the rights and freedoms of health workers. Furthermore, migration of health personnel not only emphasized contradictory relations between state and profession, but also exposed a conflict between governmental obligations to protect public health and international treaties designed to secure individual freedoms such as freedom to movement and choice of employment (WHO 2002).

The problem of effective regulation has been also discussed in relation to the labor rights of foreign health workers in the country of destination: for example, rights to just and favorable conditions of work and protection from occupational and racial discrimination, to social benefits coverage, and to representation in professional associations and trade unions (Kingma 2006; Smith et al. 2006). The vulnerability of migrant health workers is exploited by some private recruitment agencies, which engage in illegal and unethical practices such as charging recruitment fees; providing misleading information about the nature and location of a job or about working and living conditions; and employing coercive recruitment practices, like withholding travel documents, debt bondage, and threats (UNODC 2015).

Finally, another dimension of the perceived regulatory problem of health worker migration concerns patient safety in destination countries. It raises the question of how to ensure that the professional qualifications and language proficiency of foreign health workers conform to national standards. Although there are professional organizations that monitor the skills of international health workers, the coherence of education systems and professional standards across the world remains a concern. For instance, the original version of the EU Directive on the Recognition of Professional Qualifications (Directive 2005/36/EC 2005), which allowed professionals, including health workers, educated in the EU region to bypass the national supervisory bodies, caused concerns among national professional organizations and healthcare practitioners regarding patient safety (Royal College of Nursing 2011). These criticisms propelled a review of the implementation of this directive that resulted in its amended version (Directive 2013/55/EU 2013).[3]

As revealed above, the effective regulation of health worker mobility poses a number of questions, such as how to protect the right to health in source countries; how to ensure coherence of professional qualifications of foreign health workers with national standards, particularly when mutual recognition of qualifications is promoted at the international level; and how to respect the right to freedom of movement, free choice of employment, and labor rights of migrant health workers. To sum up, migration of health personnel involves and affects many stakeholders with different interests; thus, the central problem facing these regulatory processes is how to manage migration without compromising either the rights of patients and health workers or the needs of the national health systems in both source and destination countries.

Policy Tools in the Regulation of Health Worker Migration: An Overview and the UK Case Study

A number of regulatory measures have been proposed in response to tensions invoked by the migration of health workers. These tools can be classified using various rationales, including their purpose (e.g., measures restricting or facilitating the mobility of health workers, tools protecting the rights of foreign health workers, programs for return migration, instruments for regulating recruitment agencies), the level of implementation (local, national, international, and global), and the legal status ("hard," or legally binding, and "soft," or recommendatory, tools). Figure 6.1 offers an overview of these policy tools at different levels with relevant examples.

One of the key actors in governing migration of health workers remains a nation-state that holds the primary responsibility for protecting the right to health and ensuring the availability of health services for its citizens (OHCHR 2008). Depending on political and economic contexts, both destination and source countries either impede or encourage migration of health workers. To regulate inflows of health workers from overseas, destination countries, for instance, employ an array of tools, including investment in training of the national workforce, immigration rules, professional and language standards, and ethical recommendations for employers recruiting from overseas (Young 2011). At the other end of the migratory

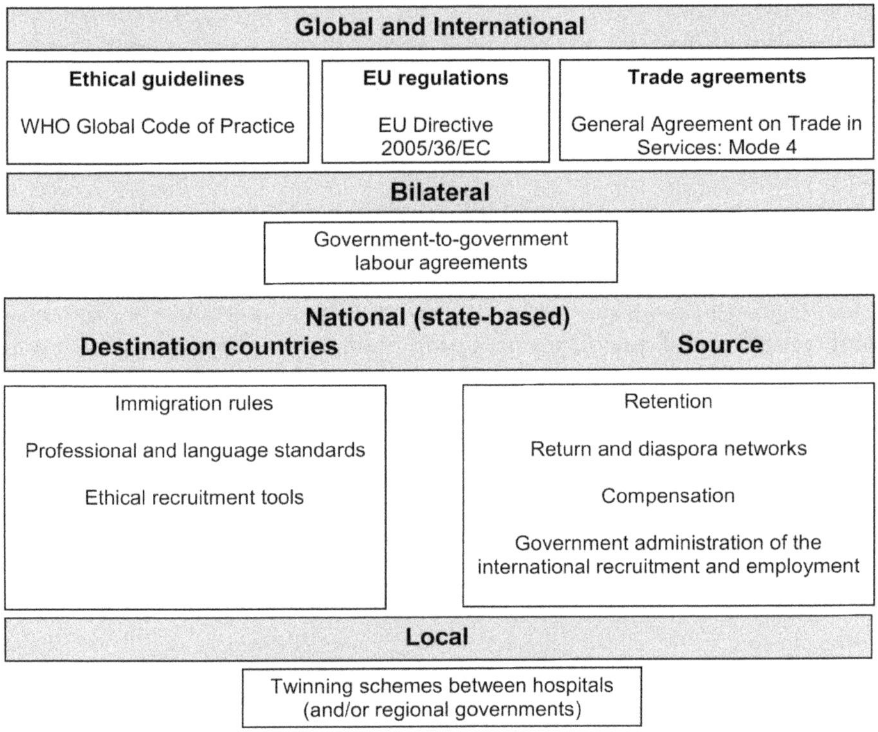

Figure 6.1 Governance framework for the regulation of cross-border health worker mobility. Figure created by the author.

process, source countries develop programs facilitating return migration (Haour-Knipe and Davies 2008); employ retention policies such as increasing wages and improving working conditions; and introduce restrictive measures, including compulsory service requirements ("bonding" schemes) and the education of particular types of health workers, who will have limited prospects for migrating overseas (Dolea 2009). Also, many source countries strongly advocate the introduction of compensatory policies also known as reparations (Gish and Godfrey 1979; Clark et al. 2006).[4] Finally, some states adopt measures to facilitate employment of home-educated health workers abroad. For instance, the Philippines stands out, as an exceptional example where the "export" of labor is institutionalized at the state level (Imson 2006). The government of the Philippines adopted an international labor migration policy in 1974 as a temporary, stopgap measure to ease unemployment, economic stagnation, and poverty. Gradually, this short-term practice was transformed into an institutionalized policy of deploying workers abroad. This culminated in the Migrant Workers and Overseas Filipinos Act, introduced in 1995 to institutionalize the principles of overseas workers' deployment and to establish a system that could protect the welfare of Filipino workers abroad. This case illustrates the ambivalent position of some source countries toward international migration of health workers. One can argue that, driven by economic pressures, such countries choose to facilitate the overseas employment of health workers and thus support their human right to freedom of movement and free choice of employment. However, such policies could also be criticized as damaging the national health system and deteriorating the access to health of those who remain in the country.

The next level in regulation of cross-border labor mobility is represented by bilateral mechanisms, including such tools as joint commissions on labor, round table meetings, and working groups between government officials in two countries (Baruah 2003; Buchan and Dovlo 2004). Often, such government-to-government agreements include twinning schemes (see Figure 6.1) deployed at the local level to facilitate cooperation and assist in the mobility of health workers between medical institutions and/or regions within two countries (Glinos 2011).[5]

At the global level, one of the most prominent regulatory tools relevant to the migration of health workers is the WHO Code of Practice on the International Recruitment of Health Personnel (WHO 2010).[6] The Code, adopted in 2010, is voluntary in nature and serves "as a reference for Member States in establishing or improving the legal and institutional framework required for the international recruitment of health personnel" (WHO 2010). Its twofold objective is to discourage the active recruitment of health personnel from developing countries that face critical shortages of health workers and to promote and disseminate best practices in sustainable health workforce planning and international recruitment.

At the level of global regions, EU regulations exemplify a distinctive case of binding mechanisms securing the right to freedom of movement and recognition of health professional qualifications.[7] Other mechanisms affecting migration of health workers at the global level are incorporated in multilateral and regional trade agreements, such as the General Agreement on Trade in Services (GATS) and the North American Free Trade Agreement (NAFTA). However, it is argued that, until now, these trade agreements have had limited overall impact on cross-border mobility of health workers (Merkur 2014). Trade agreements focus primarily on creating frameworks for recognizing professional qualifications and strengthening equivalence of professional education within global regions (Bach 2003). There is an acknowledged need for further research on possible adverse implications of trade agreements for health systems and, in particular, for the health workforce, especially within source countries (WHO Regional Office for Europe 2008).

Further, this section explores how some of these policy tools were deployed in the UK to regulate both the inflow of foreign nurses over the last fifteen years and the discourse of an unethical recruitment of foreign health workers. Since the early 2000s, the British National Health Service (NHS) has experienced a "boom and bust" cycle in the recruitment of foreign nurses (see Figure 6.2). In the early 1990s, the Conservative government in the UK considerably reduced the number of training places for nurses, and by the end of the decade, the staffing shortages in Britain had already become apparent (Buchan and Edwards 2000). In response, apart from improved retention and increased investment in education of the national health workforce, an active recruitment of nurses from abroad was deployed by the British health sector. To facilitate this inflow of foreign health personnel, a number of measures were introduced, including favorable rules for immigration and professional registration, and negotiation of bilateral arrangements with source countries in Europe and beyond.[8] Countries in sub-Saharan Africa, south Asia, and southeast Asia became primary destinations for private recruiters and NHS employers. According to Nursing and Midwifery Council data, over twenty-four thousand nurses from the Philippines, ten thousand nurses from India, and more than nine thousand nurses from South Africa were admitted to the UK professional register from 1998 to 2005 (NMC 2005). The practice of active recruitment soon emerged in public discourse as unethical policy that contributed to the critical shortage of health professionals in less developed countries. This discontent was expressed by a number of stakeholders at the international and national levels, including professional organizations and trade unions in both the UK and source countries (Plotnikova 2011). To respond to these criticisms, in 2001 the Department of Health developed the UK Code of Practice (Young 2011). The Code, which set standards and promoted best practices for NHS employers in the ethical recruitment of health workers, included recognition of the negative impact of active international recruitment on developing countries, provided guidance on international recruitment for employers, and listed countries that should not be targeted with active recruitment campaigns. Then, in 2003, jointly with the Department for International Development (DFID), the Department of Health produced a list of developing countries in which shortages of health workers had reached a significant level. As a result, NHS employers were not allowed to target those countries with active recruitment campaigns. As Figure 6.2 shows, the number of foreign nurses fell sharply from 2001 to 2003. However, it is difficult to confidently associate this decline with introduction of the Code. In fact, the performance of the UK Code of Practice was publicly debated, with numerous critics arguing that it failed as a tool to stem the outflow of health workers from source countries (Mesquita and

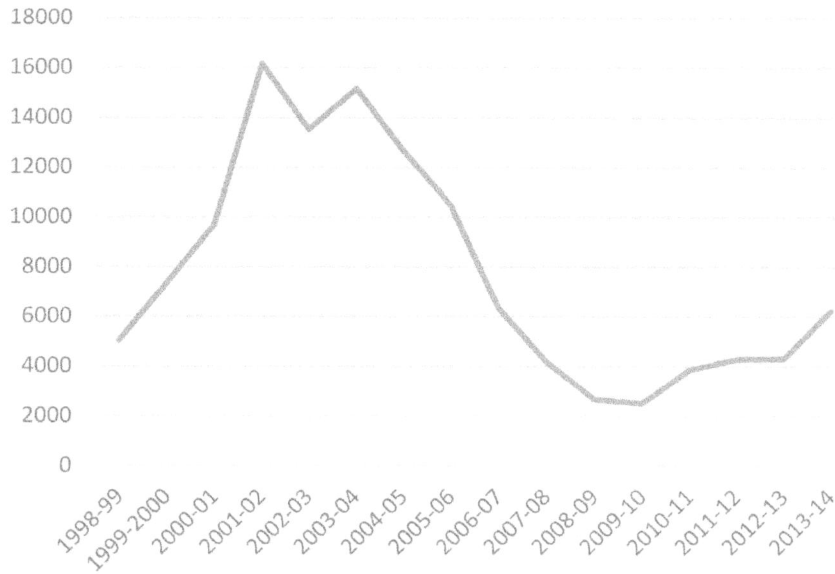

Figure 6.2 NMC initial registrations of migrant nurses (overseas and EEA), 1998–99 to 2013–14. Figure created by the author.

Gordon 2005; Mensah, Mackintosh, and Henry 2005; Martineau and Willetts 2006).

Another peak in recruitment of foreign nurses followed, in 2003–2004. At that time a revised version of the Code was produced that encouraged private agencies to subscribe to ethical recruitment principles (Department of Health 2004). From 2005 onwards, there was a consistent decrease in recruitment of overseas nurses (Figure 6.2). This was attributed largely to changes in the UK labor market for nurses, which had reached its saturation point, and many British newly qualified nurses were not able to find jobs in public sector (Guardian, 9 November 2005, https://www.theguardian.com/society/2005/nov/09/health.uknews).

Thus, the policy priority changed from encouraging to controlling the inflow of nurses from overseas (Buchan et al. 2008). Starting in 2005, a number of restrictive immigration rules and financial and administrative measures were performed (see Table 6.1).

From 2010, the number of foreign nurses on the NMC register started to increase again, with a more confident growth taking place from 2013 (Figure 6.2). To a certain extent, this was a result of the reduced national intake of nurse students in 2010 implemented by the UK coalition government, a policy pattern reminiscent to the early 1990s. From 2012 onward, UK media outlets as well as professional organizations pointed to emerging

Table 6.1 Changes to the foreign nurse registration process, immigration rules, and employment requirements since 2005

Year	Selected policy measures to curb international nurse recruitment
2005	Nursing and Midwifery Council (NMC) increases registration fee for foreign nurses
	International nurses are required to complete a twenty-day training program (the Overseas Nurses Programme, or ONP)
2006	Band 5 and 6 nursing posts are removed from the Home Office SOL
2007	NMC raises the English-language test requirements for foreign nurses
2008	Introduction of the Points-Based System (PBS) for work permits
2010	Immigration cap introduced
2011	Migration Advisory Committee (MAC) recommends limiting the group of nursing specialties included in the SOL
2012	UK Borders Agency (UKBA) increases requirements for personal funds of foreigners applying under the Tier 2 category

Sources: MAC, UKBA, and RCN (adapted from Plotnikova 2013).

shortages in medical professionals and nurses (Royal College of Nursing 2015). In 2016, nurses were added to the Shortage Occupation List (SOL) following a report by the Migration Advisory Committee that provided evidence of a recurring shortage of nurses (MAC 2016).[9] This indicated a policy shift possibly toward another period of international recruitment in the near future.

Discussion

The contemporary regulatory framework for managing the migration of health workers comprises many layers of regulation at national, bilateral, regional, and international levels, reflecting the complexity of involved interests and the diversity of existing policy tools in the regulation of health worker migration. As the UK case demonstrates, destination countries employ immigration policies, professional standards, and administrative and financial measures to control the inflow of foreign health workers. Such measures are perhaps the most powerful instruments in controlling the number of migrant health workers. They focus primarily on national health security, border control, and the quality of care provided by foreign health professionals. However, they are unlikely to address broader concerns associated with the cross-border mobility of health professionals, such as abuses of migrant workers' rights and diminishing access to health services for populations in source countries.

Unilateral ethical initiatives, such as the UK Code of Practice, could be seen as a positive development, aiming to mitigate violation of migrant health workers' rights. However, the enforcement of such mechanisms in the private sector remains a challenge (Buchan and Dovlo 2004). Moreover, the extent to which such tools intend to and/or actually address negative impacts of health worker migration in source countries is controversial. Meanwhile, in source countries, attempts to address these issues often lack sufficient resources and rely either on support from nonstate actors such as international organizations and NGOs or on the political will and priorities of governments in destination countries.

Although some scholars argue that the nation-state, using "hard" law mechanisms, still remains the key regulator of the global health labor market, the emergence of a global governance framework in which international agencies (such as WHO) become more visible and, some might argue, more influential in migration governance cannot be ignored (Bach 2007). The critical question is the implementation capacity of international instruments, as many (with the exception of the EU directives and trade agreements) principally have recommendatory intentions (Martineau et al. 2004; Stewart et al. 2007). Moreover, the enforcement of international "soft" law for the regulation of health worker migration remains a challenge. For instance, the first review of the implementation of the WHO Code of Practice revealed that of 193 WHO member states, only 56 reported on the progress of its implementation. The majority of these reports (40) came from the WHO Europe region (Siyam et al. 2013). It is recognized that one of the main concerns regarding implementation of the Code is insufficient engagement of key policy decision makers on health worker migration and international recruitment (Siyam et al. 2013).

The governance framework outlined above is incomplete without consideration of business interests and their impact on the pace of labor migration. International recruitment of health workers has become a highly profitable business managed by networks of private agencies (Kingma 2006). Flexible, fast, and adaptive recruitment agencies play a significant role in facilitating the migration process. Often driven by a desire to attain maximum profits, they not only bypass normative state regulations, such as immigration rules, but often ignore human rights articulated by international organizations (Kingma 2006). One of the emerging concerns in this area relates to the development of effective measures for controlling such agencies and ensuring that their activities do not impinge on the human rights of both migrant health workers and the population in source countries. Among other tools of regulation discussed in the literature is the Multistakeholder Initiative (MSI). This is a third-party certification system that brings together actors involved in overseeing the policy and practice of the international recruitment of health workers, namely, international organizations, NGOs, labor unions, employers, and recruitment firms. These actors negotiate standards for international recruitment and employment, which are then used by an appointed independent body for corporate performance evaluation (Pittman 2015). This mechanism has a tangible potential to address and possibly minimize negative effects of health worker migration, especially in relation to the protection of migrant health workers' rights and the regulation of recruitment agencies. It is argued that MSIs should be considered as a complementary measure to international and state regulations that offer strategies to ensure the enforcement of standards in international labor recruitment at local and national levels. This could be done by encouraging the active participation of key actors involved in policy and practice development in the international recruitment of health workers (Pittman 2015). Compared to international recommendations on ethical recruitment and employment of health professionals from overseas, MSI standards are more specific, are detailed, and provide market-based incentives for business to comply with. However, there are also concerns associated with this regulatory mechanism. For instance, participation of corporate actors in the negotiation of certification standards is seen as a weakness (Pittman 2015). Corporate engagement in this process exposes a conflict of interest between transnational business, which tend to push for less stringent regulatory standards, and NGOs, which aim to ensure that negotiated standards are more than yet another corporate tactic to demonstrate social responsibility.

Conclusion

It is important to highlight that the governance of health worker migration takes place in a complex environment of conflicting interests. Therefore, no single policy tool can provide a solution to all tensions produced by the international migration of health personnel. The contemporary policy debate on an adequate response to negative implications of health worker migration has focused on the improvement of sustainable national policies for the management of the health workforce in both source and destination countries (Buchan and Perfilieva 2015). Poor strategies for workforce planning and retention are seen as one of the key reasons for an excessive outflow of health professionals from source countries and their active recruitment by destination countries. There is little doubt that sustainable national health workforce planning should remain an important component of a policy solution to global health worker shortages, especially in disadvantaged global regions. However, policy attention should not be diverted from those measures that directly address issues associated with health worker migration and recruitment, such as abuses of migrant health workers' rights. While nation-states continue to play a primary role in planning, producing, and managing human resources for health, an adequate response to adverse consequences of health worker migration could be found in strengthening a dialogue and collaboration between policy actors at national, regional, and international levels. Innovative strategies, such as multistakeholder initiatives, as well as ways of effectively translating international norms and recommendations, and their implementation at national and local levels, need to be further explored in both source and destination countries.

Evgeniya Plotnikova, PhD, is a research fellow at the Global Public Health Unit (GPHU). She joined the GPHU in 2012 after she was awarded her PhD from the University of Edinburgh, where her doctoral thesis explored policy instruments in the regulation of international labor mobility in the health sector. Her research focused on the use of government-to-government agreements in the international recruitment of nurses to the UK from Spain, India, the Philippines, and South Africa. Her research interests revolve around regulation and policy tools in global health governance, with a particular focus on the cross-border mobility of health workers.

NOTES

This chapter is based on the study conducted by the author for a doctorate degree at the University of Edinburgh (2007–11).

1. The policy and research literature often uses the terms "health professionals," "healthcare professionals," and "health workers" interchangeably. For clarity of terminology, this chapter uses the term "health worker." This choice is informed by the position of the WHO (2006a) and the International Standard Classification of Occupations (ISCO) established by the International Labour Organization (ILO 2004). Based on these sources, the chapter defines health workers as all health service providers, including physicians, dentists, nurses, pharmacists, public health specialists, laboratory technicians, and other health service providers who deliver personal and nonpersonal health services. This term does not include health system workers, that is, managerial and support staff, such as health economists, managers, and planners, who are not engaged in the direct provision of health services but ensure that health systems function to attain their goals. It is also important

to mention that, based on the ISCO definition, health professionals do not include nurses, as nurses are placed in the separate category of nursing professionals.

2. The right to health in this human rights dilemma is understood as physical, information, and economic accessibility of health facilities, goods, and services (OHCHR 2008).
3. One of the changes is a language requirement for EU professionals. The first version of the Directive did not require a national regulator to verify the language proficiency of foreign-trained health workers. That was an employer's responsibility. However, the revised version requires national professional regulatory bodies—such as the Nursing Midwifery Council (NMC) in the UK, which is responsible for setting professional standards in nursing at the national level—to check the language skills of foreign-trained health workers (NMC 2016).
4. These are monetary contributions in the form of tax, tariff, or direct transaction from destination to source country for the loss of their health workers.
5. A twinning scheme is a two-way transfer of expertise and skills between health care institutions in two countries.
6. The WHO Code of Practice is not the only example of international ethical guidelines in the recruitment of health personnel. Recommendations of this type have been introduced by a number of international organizations, including the International Council of Nurses (2001) position statement on ethical recruitment, the World Medical Association (2003) Statement on Ethical Guidelines for the International Migration of Health Workers, and the Commonwealth Code of Practice for the International Recruitment of Health Workers (Commonwealth Secretariat 2003).
7. The regulation of labor migration within the European Union is a distinctive case. EU citizens are granted the fundamental right to freedom of movement. The free movement of workers in particular is laid down in Article 39 EC and further developed in Regulation 1612/68 (Council of the European Communities 1968); the latter provides for the right of EU citizens to work in another member state as an employee or civil servant. Another important instrument at the EU level that concerns the regulation of health worker migration is the EU directive on recognition of professional qualifications (Directive 2005/36/EC 2005; Directive 2013/55/EU 2013). In addition to these regulations, from January 2016 the European Professional Card (EPC) was made available for three categories of health workers: general care nurses, physiotherapists, and pharmacists. The EPC is an electronic certificate that is a part of the online procedure for recognition of professional qualifications (European Commission 2016).
8. In 2000, the UK government included general nursing on the Shortage Occupation List (SOL) to speed up nurse recruitment from abroad. The SOL is the resident labor market test, which allows employers to recruit foreign labor only for vacancies that were advertised for a certain period of time and were not filled by suitably skilled native candidates. However, if the profession is listed on the SOL, which specifies occupations that are in high demand, employers are not required to com-

plete a resident labor market test. For instance, in the UK this period should not be less than twenty-eight calendar days (NHS Employers 2017).

9. The Migration Advisory Committee is an independent public body that advises the government on migration issues (MAC 2016).

REFERENCES

Bach, S. 2003. "International Migration of Health Workers: Labour and Social Issues." Working Paper WP.209, Sectorial Activities Programme. International Labour Office, Geneva, July. Retrieved 3 April 2018 from http://www.rctfi.org/resources/ILO.pdf.

———. 2007. "Going Global? The Regulation of Nurse Migration in the UK." *British Journal of Industrial Relations* 45(2): 383–403.

Baruah, N. 2003. "Bilateral Labour Agreements for Managing Migration." Geneva: International Organization for Migration.

Baumann, A., J. Blythe, C. Kolotylo, and J. Underwood. 2004. *The International Nursing Labour Market Report.* Building the Future: An Integrated Strategy for Nursing Human Resources in Canada. Ottawa: Nursing Sector Study Corporation. Retrieved 30 March 2018 from https://cna-aiic.ca/~/media/cna/page-content/pdf-fr/international_nursing_labour_market_e.pdf.

Blitz, B. K. 2005. "'Brain Circulation': The Spanish Medical Profession and International Medical Recruitment in the United Kingdom." *Journal of European Social Policy* 15(4): 363–79. doi:10.1177/0958928705057279.

Bourgain, A., P. Pieretti, and B. Zou. 2008. "The Shortage of Medical Workers in Sub-Saharan Africa and Substitution Policy." Working Paper. Retrieved 30 March 2018 from https://pub.uni-bielefeld.de/publication/2315819.

Buchan, J., and D. Dovlo. 2004. *International Recruitment of Health Workers to the UK: A Report for DFID.* London: DFID (Department for International Development) Health Systems Resource Centre. Retrieved 30 March 2018 from http://www.equinetafrica.org/sites/default/files/uploads/documents/BUChres310108.pdf.

Buchan, J., and N. Edwards. 2000. "Nursing Numbers in Britain: The Argument for Workforce Planning." *BMJ (Clinical Research Ed.)* 320(7241): 1067–70.

Buchan, J., S. Baldwin, and M. Munro. 2008. "Migration of Health Workers: The UK Perspective to 2006." OECD (Organisation for Economic Co-operation and Development) Health Working Paper No. 38. Directorate for Employment, Labour and Social Affairs, OECD, 13 October. Retrieved 30 March 2018 from http://www.who.int/hrh/migration/Case_study_UK_2008.pdf.

Buchan, J., I. Seccombe, and R. Hutt. 2006. *Nurse Migration and the Commonwealth.* London: Commonwealth Secretariat.

Buchan J., and G. Perfilieva. 2015. "Making Progress towards Health Workforce Sustainability in the WHO European Region." Copenhagen: WHO Regional Office for Europe.

Campbell, J., G. Dussault, J. Buchan, F. Pozo-Martin, M. Guerra Arias, C. Leone, A. Siyam, and G. Cometto. 2014. *A Universal Truth: No Health without a Workforce.* Geneva: Global Health Workforce Alliance, World Health Organization. Retrieved 30 March 2018 from http://www.who.int/workforcealliance/knowledge/resources/GHWA-a_universal_truth_report.pdf.

Clark, P. F., J. B. Stewart, and D. A. Clark. 2006. "The Globalization of the Labour Market for Health-Care Professionals." *International Labour Review* 145(1/2): 37–64.

Commonwealth Secretariat. 2003. *Commonwealth Code of Practice for the International Recruitment of Health Workers.* Retrieved 3 April 2018 from https://www.odi.org/sites/odi.org.uk/files/odi-assets/events-documents/2440.pdf.

Council of the European Communities. 1968. *Regulation (EEC) No 1612/68 of the Council of 15 October 1968 on Freedom of Movement for Workers within the Community.* Retrieved 3 April 2018 from http://eur-lex.europa.eu/legal-content/HR/TXT/?uri=CELEX:31968R1612.

de Mesquita, J. B., and M. Gordon. 2005. "The International Migration of Health Workers: A Human Rights Analysis." London: Medact. Retrieved 3 April 2018 from http://www.equinetafrica.org/sites/default/files/uploads/documents/BUEhres.pdf.

Department of Health. 2004. *Code of Practice for the International Recruitment of Healthcare Professionals.* Leeds, UK: Department of Health. Retrieved 3 April 2018 from http://webarchive.nationalarchives.gov.uk/20130107105354/http://www.dh.gov.uk/prod_consum_dh/groups/dh_digitalassets/@dh/@en/documents/digitalasset/dh_4097734.pdf.

Dolea, C. 2009. "Increasing Access to Health Workers in Remote and Rural Areas through Improved Retention." Background paper for the first expert meeting to develop evidence-based recommendations to increase access to health workers in remote and rural areas through improved retention, Geneva, 2–4 February. Geneva: World Health Organization. Retrieved 3 April 2018 from http://www.who.int/hrh/migration/background_paper.pdf.

Dovlo, D. 2005. "Taking More Than a Fair Share? The Migration of Health Professionals from Poor to Rich Countries." *PLOS Med* 2(5): e109.

European Commission. 2012. "Commission Staff Working Document on an Action Plan for the EU Health Workforce." Retrieved 3 April 2018 from http://ec.europa.eu/health/workforce/docs/staff_working_doc_healthcare_workforce_en.pdf.

———. 2016. "Free Movement of Professionals." Retrieved 3 April 2018 from http://ec.europa.eu/growth/single-market/services/free-movement-professionals_en.

Galvez-Tan, J. 2005. "Philippines: The Challenge of Managing Migration, Retention and Return of Health Professionals." Powerpoint Presentation at the Academy for Health Conference, New York.

Gish, O., and M. Godfrey. 1979. "A Reappraisal of the 'Brain Drain'—With Special Reference to the Medical Profession." *Social Sciences & Medicine* 13(1): 1–11.

Glinos, I.A. 2011. "Cross-Border Collaboration." In *Cross-Border Health Care in the European Union: Mapping and Analysing Practices and Policies,* ed. M. Wismar, W. Palm, J.

Figueras, K. Ernst, and E. van Ginneken, 217–255. Copenhagen: European Observatory on Health Systems and Policies. Retrieved 3 April 2018 from http://www.euro.who.int/__data/assets/pdf_file/0004/135994/e94875.pdf.

Haour-Knipe, M., and A. Davies. 2008. *Return Migration of Nurses*. Geneva: International Centre on Nurse Migration. Retrieved 3 April 2018 from http://www.intlnursemigration.org/wp-content/uploads/2014/10/ReturnmigrationA4.pdf.

ILO (International Labour Organization). 2004. "Minor Group 222: Health Professionals (except Nursing." *ISCO: International Standard Classification of Occupations*. Retrieved 3 April 2018 from http://www.ilo.org/public/english/bureau/stat/isco/isco88/222.htm.

Imson, M. 2006. "Managing the Mobility of Health Workers: The Philippine Experience." Migration and Human Resources for Health, International Conference Center, Geneva, 23 March. Retrieved 3 April 2018 from http://www.iom.int/migration-and-human-resources-health-2006.

International Council of Nurses. 2001. "Ethical Nurse Recruitment." Position Statement. Retrieved 3 April 2018 from http://www.icn.ch/images/stories/documents/publications/position_statements/C03_Ethical_Nurse_Recruitment.pdf.

Johnson, T. 1995. "Governmentality and the Institutionalisation of Expertise." In *Health Professions and the State in Europe*, ed. T. Johnson, G. Larkin, and M. Saks, 7–24. London: Routledge.

Kingma, M. 2006. *Nurses on the Move: Migration and the Global Health Care Economy*. Ithaca, NY: Cornell University Press.

Kline, D.S. 2003. "Push and Pull Factors in International Nurse Migration." *Journal of Nursing Scholarship* 35(2): 107–11.

Lorenzo, F.M.E., J. Galvez-Tan, K. Icamina, and L. Javier. 2007. "Nurse Migration from a Source Country Perspective: Philippine Country Case Study." *Health Services Research* 42(3 Pt. 2): 1406–18. doi:10.1111/j.1475-6773.2007.00716.x.

MAC (Migration Advisory Committee). 2016. *Partial Review of the Shortage Occupation List: Review of Nursing*. London: Migration Advisory Committee. Retrieved 3 April 2018 from https://www.gov.uk/government/uploads/system/uploads/attachment_data/file/510630/Partial_review_of_the_shortage_occupation_list_-_review_of_nursing.pdf.

Martineau, T., and A. Willetts. 2006. "The Health Workforce: Managing the Crisis Ethical International Recruitment of Health Professionals: Will Codes of Practice Protect Developing Country Health Systems?" *Health Policy* 75(3): 358–67. doi:10.1016/j.healthpol.2005.04.012.

Martineau, T., K. Decker, and P. Bundred. 2004. "'Brain Drain' of Health Professionals: From Rhetoric to Responsible Action." *Health Policy* 70(1): 1–10.

Mejia, A. 1978. "Migration of Physicians and Nurses: A World Wide Picture." *International Journal of Epidemiology* 7(3): 207–15. doi:10.1093/ije/7.3.207.

Mensah, K., M. Mackintosh, and L. Henry. 2005. "The 'Skill Drain' of Health Professionals from the Developing World: A Framework for Policy Analysis." London: Medact. Retrieved 3 April 2018 from http://www.medact.org/wp-content/uploads/2014/03/2.-the-skills-drain-of-health-professionals.pdf.

Merkur, S. 2014. "Policy Responses Facilitating Mobility or Mitigating Its Negative Effects: National, EU and International Instruments." In *Health Professional Mobility in a Changing Europe: New Dynamics, Mobile Individuals and Diverse Responses,* vol. 2, ed. J. Buchan, M. Wismar, I. A. Glinos, and J. Bremner, 301–325. Copenhagen. Retrieved 3 April 2018 from http://www.euro.who.int/__data/assets/pdf_file/0006/248343/Health-Professional-Mobility-in-a-Changing-Europe.pdf.

Ncayiyana, D. 1999. "Doctor Migration Is a Universal Phenomenon." *South African Medical Journal* 89(11): 1107.

NMC (Nursing and Midwifery Council). 2005. *Statistical Analysis of the Register.* London: NMC.

———. 2016. "English Language Requirements." Retrieved 3 April 2018 from https://www.nmc.org.uk/registration/joining-the-register/trained-outside-the-eueea/ielts/.

NHS Employers. 2017. "Shortage Occupation List". Retrieved 3 April 2018 from http://www.nhsemployers.org/your-workforce/recruit/employer-led-recruitment/international-recruitment/shortage-occupation-list.

OECD (Organisation for Economic Co-operation and Development). 2004. "The International Mobility of Health Professionals: An Evaluation and Analysis Based on the Case of South Africa." In *Trends in International Migration,* Part 3, 115–51. Paris: OECD. Retrieved 3 April 2018 from https://www.oecd.org/migration/mig/37965326.pdf.

———. 2010. "International Migration of Health Workers: Improving International Co-operation to Address the Global Health Workforce Crisis." *OECD Policy Brief,* February. Retrieved 3 April 2018 from https://www.oecd.org/migration/mig/44783473.pdf.

———. 2016. "Focus on Health Workforce Policies in OECD Countries: Right Jobs, Right Skills, Right Places." OECD, March. Retrieved 3 April 2018 from http://www.oecd.org/health/health-systems/Health-workforce-policies-in-oecd-countries-Policy-brief.pdf.

OHCHR (Office of the United Nations High Commissioner for Human Rights). 2008. "The Right to Health." Fact Sheet No. 31. United Nations, Geneva, June. Retrieved 3 April 2018 from http://www.ohchr.org/Documents/Publications/Factsheet31.pdf.

Pittman, P. 2015. "Alternative Approaches to the Governance of Transnational Labor Recruitment." *International Migration Review* 50(2): 269–314.

Plotnikova, E. 2011. "Recruiting Foreign Nurses for the UK: The Role of Bilateral Labour Agreements." PhD thesis, Edinburgh: University of Edinburgh.

———. 2013. "The Recruitment of Foreign Nurses in the UK: Exploring Shifts over the Last 15 Years." *Journal of Siberian Federal University: Humanities and Social Sciences* 8(6): 1205–18.

Robinson, S., and P. Griffiths. 2007. *Nursing Education and Regulation: International Profiles and Perspectives.* London: National Nursing Research Unit. Retrieved 3 April 2018 from http://eprints.soton.ac.uk/348772/1/NurseEduProfiles.pdf.

European Commission. 2011. "Green Paper on Modernising the Professional Qualifications Directive (Directive 2005/36/EC)." Retrieved 3 April 2018 from http://eur-lex.europa.eu/LexUriServ/LexUriServ.do?uri=COM:2011:0367:FIN:en:PDF.

———. 2015. "Frontline First: The Fragile Frontline." London: Royal College of Nursing. Retrieved 3 April 2018 from http://royalnursing.3cdn.net/9808b89b8bfd137533_krm6b9wz7.pdf.

Siyam, A., P. Zurn, O. C. Ro, G. Gedik, K. Ronquilo, C. J. Co, C. Vaillancourt-Laflamme, J. dela Rosa, G. Perfilieva, and M. R. Dal Poz. 2013. "Monitoring the Implementation of the WHO Global Code of Practice on the International Recruitment of Health Personnel." *Bulletin of the World Health Organization* 91(11): 816–23.

Smith, P. A., H. Allan, L.W. Henry, J. A. Larsen, and M. M. Mackintosh. 2006. *Valuing and Recognising Talents of a Diverse Healthcare Workforce.* REOH Study. Retrieved 3 March 2018 from https://matrix.rcn.org.uk/__data/assets/pdf_file/0008/78713/003078.pdf.

Stewart, J., D. Clark, and P. Clark. 2007. "Migration and Recruitment of Health Professionals: Causes, Consequences and Policy Responses." *Focus Migration.* Policy Brief 7. Hamburg Institute of International Economics, August. Retrieved 3 April 2018 from http://www.hwwi.org/uploads/tx_wilpubdb/PB07_Health.pdf.

Stilwell, B. 2009. "Cause for Concern: The Global Health Workforce and the State of Our Health." Retrieved 3 March 2011 from http://globalhealth.washington.edu/media/gallery/4680.

UN (United Nations) General Assembly. 1948. *Universal Declaration of Human Rights,* 10 December, 217 A (III). Retrieved 3 April 2018 from http://www.un.org/en/universal-declaration-human-rights/.

UNCESCR (United Nations Committee on Economic, Social and Cultural Rights). 2000. *General Comment No. 14: The Right to the Highest Attainable Standard of Health (Art. 12 of the Covenant),* 11 August, E/C.12/2000/4. Retrieved 3 April 2018 from http://www.refworld.org/docid/4538838d0.html.

UNODC (United Nations Office on Drugs and Crime). 2015. *The Role of Recruitment Fees and Abusive and Fraudulent Recruitment Practices of Recruitment Agencies in Trafficking in Persons.* Vienna: UNODC. Retrieved 3 April 2018 from https://www.unodc.org/documents/human-trafficking/2015/Recruitment_Fees_Report-Final-22_June_2015_AG_Final.pdf.

WHO (World Health Organization). 2002. *25 Questions and Answers on Health and Human Rights.* Health and Human Rights Publication Series Issue No. 1 (July). Geneva: WHO. Retrieved 3 April 2018 from http://www.who.int/hhr/NEW37871OMSOK.pdf.

———. 2006a. "The Global Shortage of Health Workers and Its Impact." Fact Sheet No. 02, Geneva: WHO.

———. 2006b. *The World Health Report 2006: Working Together for Health.* Geneva: WHO. Retrieved 3 April 2018 from http://www.who.int/whr/2006/whr06_en.pdf.

———. 2010. "WHO Global Code of Practice on the International Recruitment of Health Personnel." Retrieved 26 October 2016 from http://www.who.int/hrh/migration/code/WHO_global_code_of_practice_EN.pdf.

———. 2016a. *Global Strategy on Human Resources for Health: Workforce 2030.* Draft 1.0. Geneva: WHO. Retrieved from http://www.who.int/hrh/resources/global_strategyHRH.pdf.

———. 2016b. "Density per 1,000: Data by Country." *Global Health Observatory Data Repository.* Retrieved 26 October 2016 from http://apps.who.int/gho/data/node.main.A1444.

WHO Executive Board. 2004. "Recruitment of Health Workers from the Developing World: Report by the Secretariat." EB114/5, 19 April. Geneva: WHO. Retrieved 3 April 2018 from http://apps.who.int/iris/bitstream/10665/20165/1/B114_5-en.pdf.

WHO Regional Office for Europe. 2008. *Recruitment and Retention of Health Workers' Policy Options towards Global Solidarity.* Copenhagen: WHO. Retrieved 3 April 2018 from http://www.euro.who.int/__data/assets/pdf_file/0003/103872/E91417.pdf.

World Medical Association. 2003. "WMA Statement on Ethical Guidelines for the International Migration of Health Workers." Retrieved 3 April 2018 from https://www.wma.net/policies-post/wma-statement-on-ethical-guidelines-for-the-international-migration-of-health-workers/.

Young, R. 2011. "A Major Destination Country: The United Kingdom and Its Changing Recruitment Policies." In *Health Professional Mobility and Health Systems: Evidence from 17 European Counties,* ed. M. Wismar, C. B. Maier, I. A. Glinos, G. Dussault, J. Figueras, 295–337. Copenhagen: European Observatory on Health Systems and Policies. Retrieved 3 April 2018 from http://apps.who.int/iris/bitstream/10665/170421/1/Health-Professional-Mobility-Health-Systems.pdf.

Zurn, P., M. R. Dal Poz, B. Stilwell, and O. Adams. 2004. "Imbalance in the Health Workforce." *Human Resources for Health* 2: 13.

PART III

Patient Navigation and Mobile Technologies of Care

Ginger A. Johnson

> By default, modern medicine will have to become increasingly adept at managing inequality rather than managing (providing) care.
>
> —Barbara Rylko-Bauer and Paul Farmer, "Managed Care or Managed Inequality?"

The four chapters presented in this section describe health interventions tailored to better reach populations for the provision of services that are accessible, understandable, contextually appropriate, culturally relevant, and confidential, and that preserve the dignity of the patients. These interventions involve the use of new and existing technologies to bring patients and providers together, from the innovative use of a smartphone app in an emerging economy that has made recent (and pivotal) political movements away from decades of isolationist policy, to the deployment of mobile "healthcare train" clinics by using the largest rail infrastructure on the African continent. Within the unique geographies, populations, and health conditions described in this section, the authors remind us that it is not any particular form of mobility or technology that should determine how patients and providers can be better linked, but rather the historical, political, and social context of individual populations and their health needs.

The chapters in this section identify concerns that arise from the practical challenges of providing healthcare to hard-to-reach populations. As a result, innovative practices for bringing patients and providers together are innovative not necessarily because they rely on any particular technology—

new or otherwise—but because they identify the needs of individual populations and their unique challenges in accessing care. As Pols (2012: 145) points out, the technological applications of telecare (i.e., "care at a distance") do not mean that "innovative care practices are . . . anarchistic practices that go in just any direction as long as the innovation runs," but instead exist on a foundation of care practices embedded within existing (and dynamic) social contexts. In a similar vein, the chapter by Engelman demonstrates that methods of reaching the deaf and hard-of-hearing in Kenya, which may now take advantage of community-led healthcare delivery and the opportunities afforded by mHealth (mobile health) and its associated innovations. By contrast, Briskin and Gallo provide a contemporary example of the launching and "rebirth" of an mHealth endeavor in Myanmar and, in so doing, remind us that any technology-driven intervention requires continual monitoring and evaluation in order to meet the changing health needs of its intended beneficiaries.

Once tackling the issue of how to bring patients and providers together, the process of knowledge translation—"a process that involves active and conscious participation of knowledge translators and knowledge recipients"—involves the translation of key health messages from "active" healthcare providers and facilitators in order to enable the "conscious participation" of their patients (Shea, Andersson, and Henry 2009: 2). For Srinivas and Paphitis, this process requires the engagement of future pharmacology professionals in service-learning activities that increase their understanding of the health needs of rural South Africans living in poverty, while also providing a valuable service in translating text-based medicine information leaflets into pictographic instructions understandable to illiterate populations. Turning to the politically challenging and culturally conservative context of the US South, the chapter by Edmiston describes the need for peer advocates to act as facilitators between transgender patients and healthcare providers in order to ensure patients can *safely* navigate their healthcare systems, while also helping clinic and hospital staff better understand the unique needs of transgender people.

All of the chapters presented here seek to find workable solutions for meeting the health needs of diverse groups of marginalized and vulnerable populations spread across three continents and four countries. The programs and ideas introduced by these authors are innovative interventions that can be evaluated, modified, and expanded in order to reach the hard-to-reach, strive for health equity, and challenge the stasis of the status quo.

Discussion Questions

In reading through the chapters in this section, it may be useful to keep the following questions in mind:

1. What inequalities in healthcare access do these targeted program interventions help to overcome? What opportunities do they afford the populations they serve?
2. To what extent can community-led approaches facilitate mobility and access in healthcare delivery?
2. How is technology being used (or not) to deliver healthcare to hard-to-reach populations?
3. How might the interventions described here (and their unique contextual motivators) be applied in other contexts?

REFERENCES

Pols, Jeannette. 2012. *Care at a Distance: On the Closeness of Technology.* Amsterdam: Amsterdam University Press.

Rylko-Bauer, Barbara, and Paul Farmer. 2002. "Managed Care or Managed Inequality? A Call for Critiques of Market-Based Medicine." *Medical Anthropology Quarterly* 16(4): 476–502.

Shea, Beverly, Neil Andersson, and David Henry. 2009. "Increasing the Demand for Childhood Vaccination in Developing Countries: A Systematic Review." *BMC International Health and Human Rights* 9(Suppl. 1): S5. doi:10.1186/1472-698X-9-S1-S5.

CHAPTER 7

HIV/AIDS and Voluntary Counseling and Testing (VCT) Services for Deaf Kenyans

Alina Engelman

Disability poses a host of issues—literal and virtual—related to mobility and access to healthcare. Mobility in all its facets comes into play: social, political, and linguistic mobility; access to information and services; and the availability of communications technology. People with various disabilities have developed creative ways to navigate inaccessible environments and create new forms of mobility and economic development, as Friedner (2014) has found in India among the Deaf. Yet, communication barriers and status as a minority can impede the delivery of information and care to a Deaf community in a health crisis. However, mobilization of this community, drawing upon its strengths, can serve as an effective strategy for dealing with problems of differential mobility empowerments in a pandemic (Wohlfeiler 2002). Addressing the needs of the Deaf community in Kenya in response to HIV/AIDS serves as a case in point.[1]

The status of Deaf Kenyans as a linguistic minority and a marginalized group with a distinct identity renders them a discrete community within the larger Kenyan nation-state. This position complicates the situation of

Deaf Kenyan people living with HIV/AIDS (PLWHA). The circumstances of the estimated half-million Deaf Kenyans adds an extra dimension to Susan Sontag's (1970: 2) statement about the estrangement caused by disease: "Illness is the night-side of life, a more onerous citizenship. Everyone who is born holds dual citizenship, in the kingdom of the well and in the kingdom of the sick. Although we all prefer to use only the good passport, sooner or later each of us is obliged, at least for a spell, to identify ourselves as citizens of that other place." The relative isolation of the Deaf community in Kenya, when first faced with the HIV/AIDS crisis, stands in sharp contrast to the explosive mobility of the virus itself. Sontag's metaphor of the passport is useful in considering issues of mobility and immobility—and the potential of mHealth—for HIV/AIDS care for Deaf Kenyans. Sontag's association of passport and health, an extension of what Salazar and Smart (2011: 1) refer to as the "root metaphor" of mobility, speaks to the problematic status of HIV+ Deaf Kenyans.

In 2006, the author conducted the first qualitative needs assessment of Deaf and hard-of-hearing Kenyans receiving educational and medical HIV/AIDS services provided by Liverpool VCT Kenya (renamed LVCT Health). The research was supported by a Lindsay Fellowship for Research in Africa provided by the Yale Center for International Studies.[2] The study included focus groups of Deaf Kenyans and one-on-one interviews with Deaf Kenyans with HIV/AIDS, as well as interviews with Deaf Voluntary Counseling and Testing (VCT) staff and program directors. This study focused on the unique communication challenges faced by Deaf Kenyans navigating the AIDS crisis and noted the innovative use of mobile units as one tool for servicing the most isolated members of that community.

Now, a decade later, is a propitious time to revisit and review the status of Deaf Kenyans in the age of AIDS in light of the "mobilities turn," the theoretical development of the mobility paradigm as well as the advancement of digital technology enabling new forms of mHealth (Büscher and Urry 2009). This chapter is informed by a cultural and media studies framework that understands mobilizing healthcare in the context of a new infrastructure developed by an NGO to empower Deaf Kenyans to access HIV/AIDS treatment, education, and support. It recognizes the need for linguistically and culturally appropriate approaches to the Deaf Kenyan community—which can be hard to reach, geographically and otherwise—in keeping with the stricture of D'Andrea, Ciolfi, and Gray (2011: 150) that "mobilities deserve to be examined in their own singularity, centrality and contingent determination." A related premise is the inadequacy of mass communication informational strategies and the relevance of theories of participatory and social change communication (SCC) to empower the Deaf Kenyan community to address the AIDS pandemic. Chandwani and Gopal (2010:

24) write of this approach: "Social change communication is an umbrella term involving strategic use of advocacy, media, interpersonal and dialogue based communication, and social mobilization to systematically accelerate change in the underlying drivers of HIV risk, vulnerability and impact." Furthermore, "communication is an essential element of AIDS prevention, treatment and care efforts. Historically, such efforts have been limited by a focus on getting messages out about how HIV is transmitted, with lesser attention to cultural and social contexts in which such communication occurs" (Chandwani and Gopal 2010: 23). As this chapter will illustrate, the SCC philosophy as practiced by LVCT Health has the potential to empower the Deaf Kenyan community.

Needs Assessment Methods: Evaluating Deaf VCT Services in Kenya

In 2006, despite anecdotal evidence of the Deaf VCT program's effectiveness in educating and testing the Deaf community, further input was sought directly from Deaf Kenyans themselves. The author conducted a nationwide needs assessment and qualitative analysis that articulated the desires, ideas, perceptions, challenges, and experiences of Deaf Kenyan PLWHA, as well as employees of the Deaf VCT program, including predominately deaf VCT directors, community mobilizers, and counselors in Nairobi, Kisumu, and Mombasa. In addition, the author conducted participant observation and interviews with Deaf mobile VCT participants, teachers for the Deaf, and Deaf Kenyans who entered VCT sites asking for more information about HIV/AIDS. At a critical juncture of the program, LVCT pioneered the First Deaf National HIV/AIDS Conference in June 2006. Data were collected from focus groups at the Nyaweri Deaf VCT and the Nairobi Deaf VCT, as well as from one-on-one interviews with Deaf Kenyan PLWHA in rural areas outside of Kisumu and Mombasa. The challenges inherent in methodologies of mobility were mitigated by Deaf members of the community who also worked at LVCT Health and had an intimate understanding of the community combined with a commitment to providing services. That existing framework enabled my mobility as a Deaf researcher and access to both organizational operations as well as access to participants who had received services.

On a sweltering day in June 2006, in the Nairobi Deaf HIV/AIDS VCT Center located in the city's central business district, a focus group of Deaf Kenyans spoke openly about barriers regarding equal access to healthcare, including information and treatment in response to the HIV/AIDS pandemic. The focus group was part of a nationwide needs assessment and qualitative analysis conducted by the author regarding HIV/AIDS counseling and testing services for the Deaf community throughout Kenya (Engelman 2007). Kenyan Sign Language (KSL) was the primary language used by the participants. One focus group participant stated, "When I was pregnant in the hospital, he [the doctor] dispensed medicine that made me sick. I didn't understand what the medicine was. If I had an interpreter it wouldn't have happened." Another, sick with tuberculosis, said, "I want to go to the hospital when I am sick, but it's so hard because the hearing look at you, they don't know how to deal with you. . . . In 2005 it started, I was so sick and I felt a lot of pain; I was asking the doctors and they understood nothing." A third pointed to obstacles to health literacy and her difficulty in learning about HIV/AIDS: "I was twenty-five when I learned about it. Before 1990, in primary school, I didn't understand it. . . . The government gave out a lot of posters but a lot of them were in Kiswahili, and I did not understand them until they came up with the sign language posters."

The Deaf in Kenya face obstacles to healthcare access not just because of language barriers, however. In some instances, they are turned away from hospitals or VCT centers for testing and counseling due to the stigma of deafness and the erroneous perception that communication would not be possible. The struggle of Deaf Kenyan PLWHA to communicate with healthcare providers hinders their access to quality care, and this struggle to access healthcare has been found in other Deaf populations worldwide (Ubido, Huntington, and Warburton 2002). It can lead to misunderstandings about the importance of adherence and the dosage, frequency, and purpose of medication, denying Deaf Kenyans the benefits of progress in the development of antiretroviral (ARV) drugs. Some Deaf Kenyans even believe that such a medical regimen only serves to make them sicker. As a consequence, some Deaf PLWHA were reluctant to take ARVs even though the drugs were freely available.

Deaf people are affected by traditional cultural factors and misconceptions in Kenyan society that contribute to the HIV/AIDS epidemic. For example, the Luo ethnic group in western Kenya has customary laws surrounding marriage—namely, bride wealth, birth order, land inheritance, wife inheritance, and polygamy—that can inadvertently contribute to the spread of HIV (Sheller 2006). Myths, ignorance, and stereotypes are often propagated in an insular Deaf subculture in ways less likely to occur in Kenyan society at large. One Deaf adult interviewed for training as an HIV/AIDS community mobilizer and counselor in Kisumu made the following statement about HIV/AIDS: "You can get HIV if you put too much sugar in your tea with milk" (Opiyo, Muruka, and Engelman 2006). Some Deaf people, upon finding out that they are HIV+, think that being positive is a good thing because the sign for "positive" in reference to something good is also the sign for "plus." To be sure, misinformation persists among the general Kenyan population; however, hearing individuals have the ability to be exposed to information and perspectives via mass media that remain largely inaccessible to the Deaf. In general, Deaf people have limited access to dominant languages in hearing societies, which is where most information about health issues, including HIV, is circulated, processed, and understood. Radio, a medium of importance in Kenya, cannot be accessed by the Deaf. Television is of limited use given the paucity of captioning. Even billboards or pamphlets regarding HIV/AIDS in Kiswahili are largely ineffective for a Deaf population often afflicted by a higher rate of illiteracy than the general population.

When asked to identify the primary challenges Deaf people in Kenya faced in getting healthcare, the Nairobi focus group cited discriminatory practices resulting in increased susceptibility to illiteracy, unemployment, poverty, and isolation—especially in rural areas—as well as the overriding problem of communication. Language, together with a host of cultural, geographic, and economic factors linked to disability, represents a critical obstacle to accessing education and treatment for HIV/AIDS to Kenya's Deaf community. Kenya is a multilingual and diverse country, with over forty tribes with variations in language and dialect. Many Deaf Kenyans have only a rudimentary knowledge of the predominant language, Kiswahili. Due to financial constraints or rural isolation, some Deaf Kenyans do not have the opportunity to attend one of Kenya's sixty-four Deaf schools and learn KSL, although it is the primary language used by Deaf Kenyans (Gallaudet University n.d.). It is estimated that 30 percent of Deaf Kenyans do not attend school; those who do attend may be taught by hearing teachers with a rudimentary knowledge of sign language, using a combination of speech and sign language in the classroom (Adoyo 2007).

Organizational Background

The 2006 focus group was conducted in conjunction with an innovative nationwide nonprofit organization, LVCT Health (originally Liverpool Voluntary Counseling and Testing and Care Kenya), to provide direct HIV education, testing, and care to vulnerable populations. In 2001, the Liverpool School of Tropical Medicine in England partnered with the Kenyan Ministry of Health to establish LVCT Health as an indigenous Kenyan NGO to provide innovative testing, treatment, and educational services for HIV prevention and treatment for PLWHA. LVCT Health, based in Nairobi with 150 stand-alone VCT sites operating throughout the country, targets groups facing social barriers that increase vulnerability to HIV/AIDS, such as sex workers, drug addicts, men who have sex with men (MSM), prisoners, and

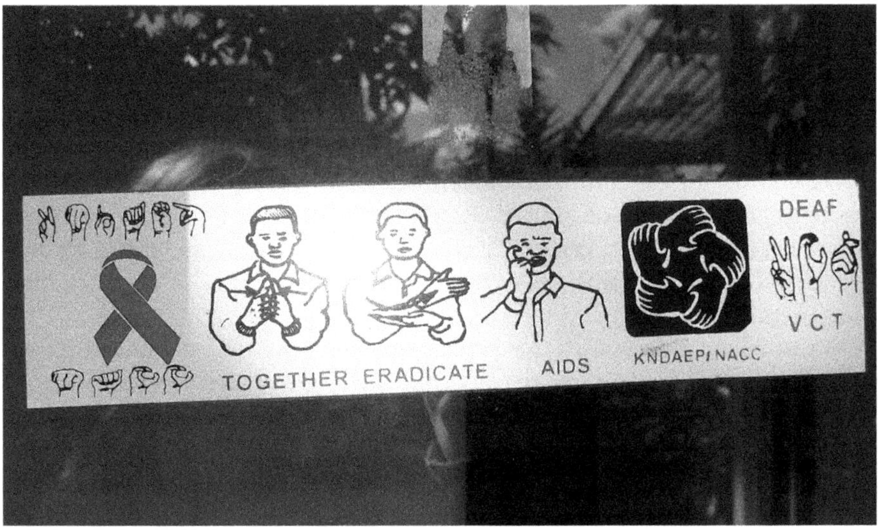

Figure 7.1 Tailor-made, accessible HIV/AIDS education message in Kenyan Sign Language (KSL) at a Deaf VCT site: "Together We Will Eradicate AIDS." 11 June 2006. Produced by the Deaf VCT Project in collaboration with the Kenya National Deaf HIV/AIDS Education Programme (KNDAEP) and the National AIDS Control Council (NACC). Photo by the author.

the approximately 1.3 million Kenyans with disabilities, including a Deaf population estimated to be as large as a half-million people.

In 2002 and 2003, LVCT Health partnered with several Deaf Kenyan organizations to inaugurate three pilot projects in Nairobi, Mombasa, and Kisumu, in which HIV testing and counseling were provided at stand-alone VCT sites in KSL. This represented the first VCT program for the Deaf in Africa. An initial published report based on the initiative concluded that "the Deaf in Kenya are at risk of HIV and there is an urgent need for Deaf-friendly HIV services, supplemented by peer education programs" (Taegtmeyer et al. 2009). LVCT Health was honored at the International AIDS Conference 2006 in Bangkok, Thailand, for its pioneering initiative and recognition of the importance of adapting HIV/AIDS programs to the needs of the Deaf (LVCT Health 2016a). LVCT Health anticipated—and contributed to—an emerging awareness of the importance of considering the HIV/AIDS crisis in relation to disability. LVCT Health played a key role in ensuring the inclusion of disability issues into Kenya's National AIDS Strategic Plan (KNASP). In 2006, UNESCO, in a report on HIV/AIDS literacy, issued a clarion call: "Meeting the HIV/AIDS prevention and care needs of persons with disability requires special attention by policy makers and program implementers at all levels" (Schenker 2005, 43).

A central feature of LVCT's program was engagement with the Kenyan Deaf community and the community's role in designing and providing services. This was in accordance with LVCT Health's "participatory and peer led approach" to serving at-risk populations (LVCT Health 2016b). The locations and programs at the three sites were developed in consultation with established Deaf organizations in the three cities, including the Kenya National Association of the Deaf (KNAD) and the Nairobi Association of the Deaf (NAD). Hearing staff at the Deaf VCT sites received basic training in KSL. However, priority was given to selecting Deaf personnel in key leadership, counseling, and community mobilization positions. For example, the director of the Deaf Program, based at the LVCT Health main office in Nairobi, was himself Deaf. Deaf Kenyans received services from Deaf directors, Deaf counselors, and Deaf community mobilizers, or from hearing staff able to communicate in KSL. Furthermore, in June 2006, LVCT Health mounted the first Deaf National HIV/AIDS Conference. Deaf leaders, organizers, and health professionals from all parts of Kenya attended. The tables were turned; the presenters were all Deaf, and the hearing needed voice interpreters to follow the proceedings.

At its three Deaf VCT sites and the national conference, LVCT Health provided a pioneering model for peer-led service delivery by and for Deaf people. LVCT Health's modus operandi—empowering and training Deaf practitioners to effectively provide counseling and treatment to their peers—marked an important step forward in the difficult task of addressing the deeply ingrained problems initially identified by the Nairobi focus group.

Pioneering Research on HIV and Deafness in the Global South

Professor Miriam Taegtmeyer of the Liverpool School of Tropical Medicine and other early associates at LVCT Health crafted a two-year project in 2004–2005 to describe and evaluate the early experience of the first organization to offer VCT services specifically for the Deaf on the African continent. Their report (Taegtmeyer et al. 2009) described the unique nature of a peer-based model of HIV services run for and by the Deaf in the developing world. It found that HIV prevalence among the Deaf at LVCT Health's three Deaf VCT sites mirrored the national rate, indicating an urgent need for Deaf HIV services, including peer education.

In a period of twenty-four months, 1,709 Deaf and 1,648 hearing clients were seen at LVCT Health sites. The rate of HIV prevalence among the Deaf VCT clients was 7 percent. That is, Deaf clients were equally at risk for HIV as their hearing counterparts—however, they were less likely to perceive themselves as being at risk, due to misunderstandings and inacces-

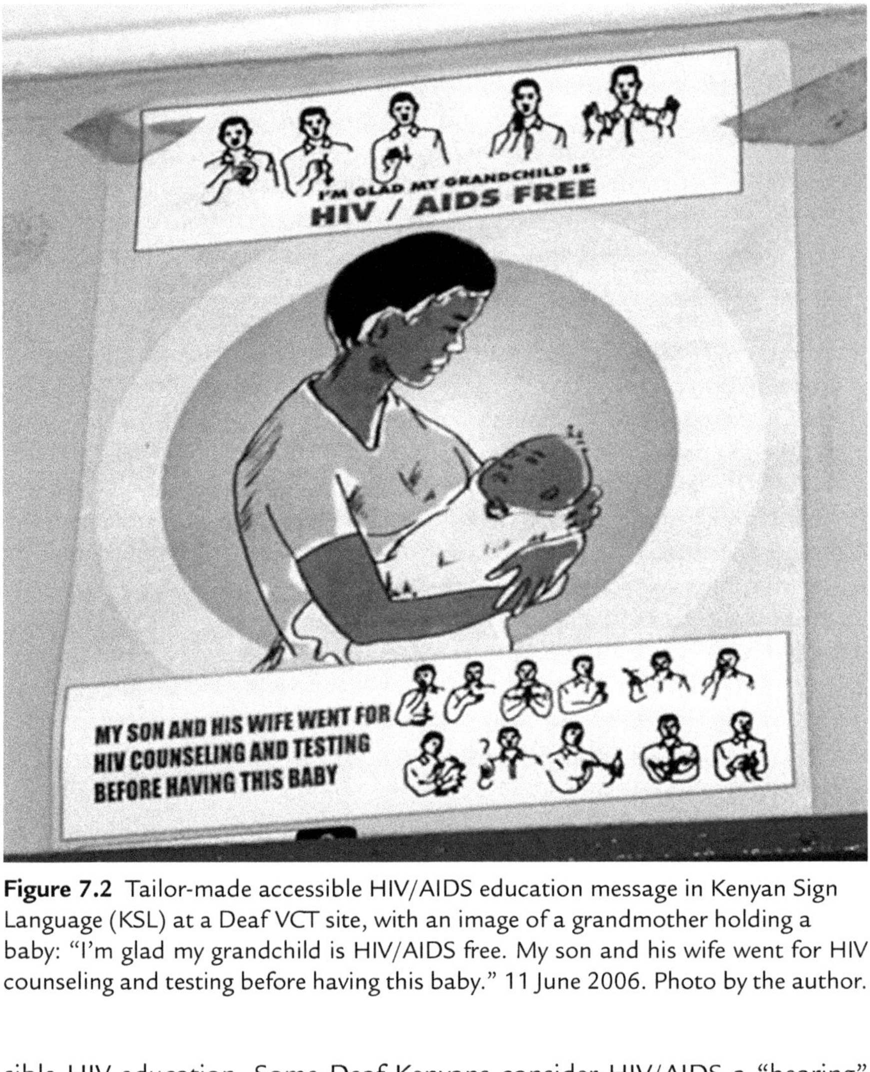

Figure 7.2 Tailor-made accessible HIV/AIDS education message in Kenyan Sign Language (KSL) at a Deaf VCT site, with an image of a grandmother holding a baby: "I'm glad my grandchild is HIV/AIDS free. My son and his wife went for HIV counseling and testing before having this baby." 11 June 2006. Photo by the author.

sible HIV education. Some Deaf Kenyans consider HIV/AIDS a "hearing" disease, perhaps due to a feeling of separation from Kenyan society at large. Nevertheless, like their hearing counterparts, Deaf clients tended to come to the VCT when they had a new partner or unprotected sex. The report emphasized the importance of the partnership between VCT services and local Kenyan Deaf organizations:

> The association of the VCT services with the local Kenyan Deaf organizations was critical to their success, and many Deaf clients expressed their appreciation of the Deaf counselors conducting both the counseling and rapid testing. This suggests that increased involvement of

> Deaf role-models and opinion leaders in national HIV/AIDS campaigns would further increase confidence in VCT as well as HIV awareness (Taegtmeyer et al. 2009: 513).

Health literacy is a key component in mobility and access to healthcare for all Deaf individuals, particularly those in the global South. According to Groce's (2006) research on HIV knowledge in Swaziland and Nigeria, the problem of low health literacy in Deaf and disabled communities is not unique to Kenya. In Swaziland, for instance, "almost all of the Deaf respondents (99 percent) reported difficulties in communicating with healthcare facility staff, which may result in less use of HIV voluntary counseling and testing services" (Groce 2006: 319).

Mobile VCT Services

Given the fact that 75 percent of Kenyans live in rural areas (World Bank 2016), in its efforts to promote health literacy and provide care, LVCT Health did not limit its outreach to its offices in Nairobi, Mombasa, and Kisumu. Deaf peer educators, relying on extensive informal community networks, reached out to Deaf churches, schools, and social organizations in the three urban centers as well. Furthermore, there was a need for peer-based VCT counselors to provide HIV education, testing, and services for Deaf Kenyans in places where geographical immobility compounded their existing problems of language and poverty. In rural areas, there are typically not enough Deaf people to form signing communities and therefore rural Deaf Kenyans may have limited access to the predominant KSL or an accessible education at a specialized school. In response, LVCT Health explored the use of mobile VCT units from the three urban sites to travel to the adjoining countryside to visit rural Deaf schools as well as to provide VCT testing and counseling at churches and community centers. LVCT Health teams tracked down and presented key health information to Deaf people in schools that were geographically isolated, and they also used these schools as staging areas for presentations to other Deaf Kenyans, who traveled from outlying areas. VCT staff traveled to rural areas via minibuses, in vans, or even by foot. In 2006, the author observed the mobile VCT teams at three schools: Kichakamkwaju Primary School, located north of the port village of Shimoni near the Tanzanian border; Reverend Muhoro School for the Deaf, in Mukurwe-ini; and Kerugoya School for the Deaf—the latter two located in the central highlands of Kenya north of Nairobi.

One particularly successful aspect of the mobile VCT operations was the use of participatory theater in rural schools for the Deaf. This tactic conformed to theater scholar Augustin Hatar's advocacy of communities

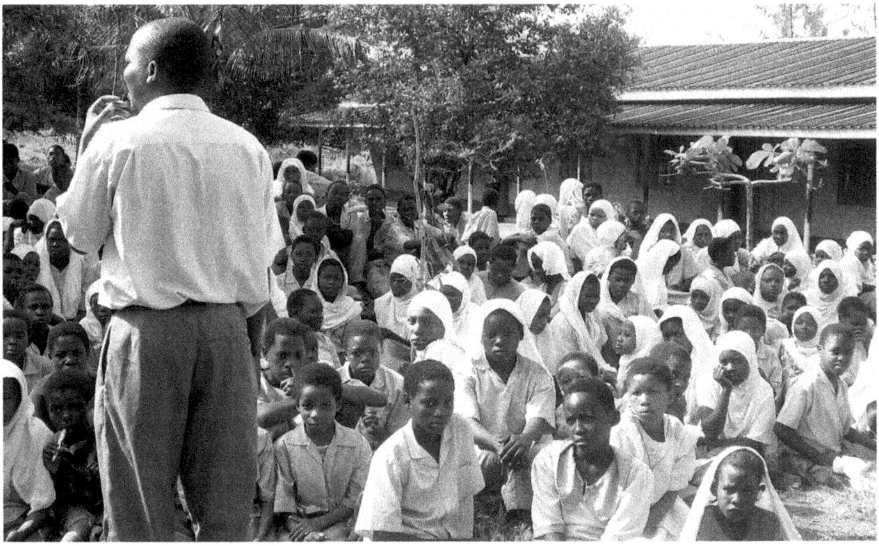

Figure 7.3 Kichakamkwaju Primary School students seated outside waiting for the participatory theater performance, in which students acted out the role of a Deaf HIV+ person, a VCT counselor, and a hearing family member. 19 July 2006. Photo by the author.

of nonprofessional actors telling their own stories. It also reflected the insights of Paulo Freire's (2000) *Pedagogy of the Oppressed* and the practices of Augusto Boal's *Theater of the Oppressed,* in which the powerless become co-creators of knowledge, seizing control of their own education as a form of empowerment. The process at Kichakamkwaju Primary School unfolded as follows: First, the Deaf peer VCT counselor educated ten to fifteen Deaf students about HIV/AIDS transmission and prevention through visual materials and KSL. The students were then asked to apply their knowledge and brainstorm to develop a skit in the classroom, to be subsequently performed in front of the entire school. In front of two hundred students and teachers, Deaf students acted out the roles of an HIV/AIDS VCT counselor, a Deaf client, and a hearing family member. The power of participatory theater was evident as the actors became animated, communicated what they had learned, and seemed to foster greater empathy toward people with HIV/AIDS. By playing the role of someone with HIV, the students were able to negotiate and connect to the experience of people living with HIV. They were asked to imagine themselves as either a stigmatized person with HIV or a person intimately connected to that person.

In addition to meeting the needs of the Deaf students, the performance was in keeping with the communication traditions of what Manyozo (2013:

38) calls "the African school, itself rooted in orality, performance, . . . and indigenous knowledge communications." A South African study of the theory and practice of entertainment education by Cardey et al (2013: 289) also makes the case for "flexibility and responsiveness to context for both development communication and HIV/AIDS communication." Further, the authors argue, "research has demonstrated that entertainment education (EE) interventions have a measurable impact on behavior in areas such as HIV/AIDS prevention" (Cardey et al. 2013: 288). Such initiatives could be expanded to include other Deaf schools, churches, and community centers in both urban and rural settings.

The mobile VCT team's use of theater represented an extension of a community-based approach to HIV/AIDS education and care. LVCT Health increased its use of mobile teams as a central tool in fulfilling its mission. In 2009, it initiated a national Deaf Mobile HIV Testing and Counseling campaign as part of an expanded use of over five hundred mobile operations targeting persons with disabilities (PWDs) throughout the nation. Since the inception of the Deaf VCT program, LVCT Health has placed increasing emphasis on not only working with people with a wide range of disabilities more broadly, but also training health counselors and what it calls "community health extension workers." As of 2016, its training institute has trained over ten thousand health workers, constituting more than 75 percent of all HIV testing and counseling personnel in the country (LVCT Health 2016c). Yet, despite LVCT Health's best efforts, there were obstacles to reaching Deaf Kenyans in remote areas. In July 2006, one mobile VCT operation in Ukunda, south of Mombasa, was well attended, but it was nonetheless limited by the fact that there were still more Deaf people in rural villages that wanted to come but could not pay for transportation.

Anne's and Jane's (Im)mobilities

Some Deaf Kenyans living with HIV who were reached by the mobile units had chosen to live in rural and less-mobile circumstances due to stigma, requiring methodologies of mobility to access their stories as well as respect for immobility. Methodologies of mobility included not only utilizing traditional transportation networks, such as *matatus* (local minibuses), but also tapping into a community network of professionals who supported the mission of empowering immobile deaf populations and who possessed extensive understanding of geographical, cultural, linguistic, and social norms and barriers. They also included learning KSL, enabling the author to communicate with and understand the community and the organizational structure. This partnership with deaf professionals was critical to tracking down Deaf Kenyans whose homes were not only in rural areas, but were also only accessible through maps of social knowledge rather than any geographical markers.

An interview with "Anne" underscored the special challenges facing Deaf Kenyans who are HIV+ living in rural areas.[3] She lived in a village far from Kisumu with no means of telecommunication, so the author and a VCT counselor took a long, bumpy ride from Kisumu in a *matatu* minibus in hopes of reaching her. Anne had previously lived in Kisumu, where a Deaf VCT staff member had not only provided her with accessible HIV testing in KSL, but also accompanied her to a hospital for management of her ARV medication. However, as a result of being cut off from the Deaf community and VCT care, she now took only vitamins. Her modest income as a caretaker was absorbed by the cost of food, and she was unable to pay for bus fare. Anne guessed at her own health status and disease progression. She estimated her CD4 counts despite the fact that it had not been tabulated in years. Her lack of mobility had a devastating effect on her ability to receive proper treatment. Furthermore, Anne's isolation was self-imposed. In 2004, she had decided to get tested at the Nyaweri Deaf VCT in Kisumu as a result of a notice at a Sunday prayer service. To Anne's mortification, the counselor who discovered she was HIV+ disclosed her status to the local Deaf community. She recalled: "People laughed at me and stopped being friends with me once they found out I was HIV+." As a result of this violation of privacy, and the stigma of the disease, Anne decided to move away, forgoing a support system and healthcare appropriate to treating her condition. A Deaf Nyaweri VCT staff member observed, "Money for the Deaf community goes to HIV/AIDS awareness but it doesn't necessarily benefit those who are HIV+. There needs to be attitudinal change" (Engelman 2006: 44).

Anne was not alone in going to great lengths to maintain secrecy. A fear of disclosure within the Deaf community also governed the actions of "Jane," an HIV+ resident of the outskirts of Mombasa.[4] When Jane decided to get tested for HIV in Kisumu, she chose to visit a hearing VCT to avoid Deaf peers. Information that would otherwise be available to her—including the meaning of her diagnosis, treatment options, follow-up care, prevention, and support—was delivered without a sign language interpreter through a spoken language she could not fully understand. The resulting communication deficit resulted in confusion about her diagnosis and adversely affected the quality of her aftercare. Jane explained that she stopped taking her ARVs because of the side effects, unaware of the availability of alternative medications with fewer side effects. Following her diagnosis, a month before this interview, she moved from Kisumu to Mombasa so that neither the Deaf community nor her family would know of her condition. A slight woman in her late teens who worked as a cook at a nearby hotel, Jane looked furtively around during the interview, fearful that she would be recognized speaking to people affiliated with LVCT Health. She was determined to avoid the risk of disclosure and gossip. She shrugged her shoulders in resignation and explained, "It won't be a problem if I die because they won't know why." Her self-exile from the Deaf community followed from her self-imposed, presumed-imminent death sentence. Unlike the Americans with Disabilities Act (1990) in the United States, there is no law in Kenya mandating sign language interpreters at VCT centers or educational institutions. There is no standard method for Deaf Kenyans to communicate in KSL with doctors or nurses other than in settings like LVCT Health that are specifically tailored to the Deaf population.

The stories of Anne and Jane reflect the propensity of many members of the Deaf community to maintain secrecy about their HIV status and suggest that the number of recorded HIV+ Deaf Kenyans may be underreported. Compounding the problem, Kenyans under the age of eighteen need parental permission to get tested. Moreover, adult Muslim women often need family permission as well. In general, Deaf culture poses special problems in regard to maintaining confidentiality. In a study of HIV/AIDS education in three residential Kenyan schools of the Deaf, Biggs (2013: 4) wrote that "participants felt that 'Deaf culture' was marked by an inability to keep secrets or that the Deaf were inherently more honest. This was in part due to the use of sign language; many teachers felt that it was impossible to have 'taboos' or keep secrets in a visual language." This feature of Deaf Kenyan culture is also underscored by Shackleton (2009: 60): "As is common in other Deaf cultures around the world, the Deaf community in Kenya becomes a second family to Deaf people. The close-knit nature of the Deaf community, commonly referred to as the Deaf 'grapevine' can make confidentiality, necessary to HIV testing, difficult to maintain." Hence, stigma reduction for PLWHA within the Deaf community should remain an integral part of promoting health literacy and providing services. In this regard, support groups for Deaf PWLHA, instituted by LVCT Health after 2006 and encouraged by the author's needs assessment, can serve as a critical tool. At the same time, increased use of digital communication technologies could be explored as a means for providing information about HIV/AIDS to the Deaf community in a more secure fashion. As suggested below, these technologies can build on the considerable achievements of LVCT Health.

A foundation official has said, "The story we need to tell of LVCT Health, which I don't think they are telling enough, is of how a small indigenous NGO has been able to occupy a space for HIV and became a leader for HIV in Kenya and even set the bar on what a good HIV program is like" (Hivos 2014: 44). LVCT Health pioneered the first VCT services for HIV/AIDS for the Deaf in Africa, among a select group of vulnerable populations. It created a viable model for providing information, counseling, and services for HIV/AIDS in Deaf communities in the developing world. Training staff in KSL was a major step in enhancing health literacy, testing, and counseling.

However, more critical to LVCT Health's development was its direct engagement with Kenya's Deaf community in planning and administering services to a linguistic and cultural minority at risk. LVCT Health avoided the pitfalls of "NGOification," which, according to Manyozo (2013), signifies top-down communication strategies advanced by Western or internationally funded NGOs. As Manyozo writes, "A key characteristic of development communication training is participatory action research, which allows collaborative learning and reflexive experience, in which development stakeholders generate knowledge and best practices together" (p. 38). Key to the success of the LVCT Health program is its guiding principles of universal access and local ownership, defined as "investment in building internal staff and institutional systems, partner organizational capacities and technical capability to promote locally led, owned and managed approaches" (LVCT Health 2014: 7). On this basis, LVCT Health, in conjunction with state and nonstate agencies, established Deaf-operated VCT sites in three major cities, supplemented by a national Deaf mobile HIV counseling and testing initiative. A report by Hivos (2014: 2) emphasized that "LVCT Health has been an advocate for inclusion of the marginalized populations in the policy and planning of responses to HIV. LVCT Health has made great inroads by building the capacity of these groups for self-agency; they are now highly empowered to push their own agendas." Hence, the process by which the Deaf community began to address HIV/AIDS in its ranks contributed to a broader capacity for empowerment. The work of LVCT Health demonstrates the benefit of tailor-made health literacy programs and post-diagnosis care in delivering care to an immobile population—and the empowering nature of community-driven healthcare delivery.

At the same time, this assessment of LVCT Health's programs concluded that "despite the successes, challenges remain. Most of the services provided to key populations especially MSM have not been integrated especially into mainstream government health facilities" (Hivos 2014: 45). This also applies to Deaf Kenyans who are HIV+. Notwithstanding groundbreaking work providing peer-led access to education, counseling, and testing in a communication-friendly environment through Deaf VCT centers, HIV treatment for the Deaf in Kenya still remains in the hands of outside agencies and hospitals that are largely ill equipped to meet the needs of Deaf and hard-of-hearing clients with HIV. Deaf VCT clients cannot receive ARV treatment or home-based care through the VCT. It is true that Deaf VCT counselors can serve as advocates and facilitators, accompanying Deaf clients with HIV to hospitals or outpatient clinics; however, these Deaf counselors are not in a position to facilitate full communication, due to the lack of sign language interpreters. Communication problems also impinge on follow-up referrals to other agencies and the quality of aftercare, increasing the risk of confusion about the benefits of ARV therapy and adherence to medication protocols. LVCT Health's peer-based HIV/AIDS education program provides critical information for individual Deaf Kenyans, but in the absence of larger legal and societal changes, such as mandatory language access at all healthcare facilities and accessible education for all Deaf Kenyans regardless of socioeconomic status, these benefits are incomplete.

The problem of stigma and privacy regarding HIV in the Deaf community feeds the immobility of Deaf PLWHA and continues to loom large, despite the advent of some Post Test Club (PTC) support groups. As use of the Internet and cell phones increases in Kenya, these technologies have the potential to serve as vehicles for delivering information and care with greater confidentiality. By 2015, approximately 70 percent of Kenyans had access to the Internet, and the rate is growing at over 10 percent a year. Of those with access, five million used Facebook (Macharia 2015). To be sure, access to the Internet is limited in poor and rural areas, which affects many members of the Deaf community. According to the World Bank (2014), in 2014 an estimated 36 percent of Kenyans did not have access to electricity. Yet, educational videos about HIV in KSL accompanied by captions could nonetheless permit increasing numbers of Deaf Kenyans to access information in private or semiprivate settings, including schools and public libraries. Steady growth in the use of smartphones and Facebook increases the ability to access videos in a mobile and fully private fashion. Video, after all, is in keeping with the visual nature of Deaf culture and enables access to visual forms of communication. Nevertheless, literacy skills are needed to navigate the Internet, which could act as a barrier to information literacy for some Deaf Kenyans. Despite these challenges, Shackleton (2009: 73) recommends wider use of educational videos, adding, "It is further recommended that Deaf persons are empowered and involved in the development of learning materials to suit their unique needs, and create a sense of ownership of future education, treatment, care and support programs." LVCT Health and others have taken steps to exploit the possibilities afforded by the Web. Sporadically, videos about HIV in KSL directed at Deaf Kenyans are posted on YouTube. For example, one video on sexual health, based on a Kenyan "Deaf Peer Education Manual," was filmed in Nairobi in 2007. On World AIDS Day in Kisumu in 2011, a video captured a short speech given by a Deaf LVCT Health program officer. It is uncertain whether there is a policy or programmatic effort to put out visual material on a regular basis. Such videos have been posted infrequently and have attracted relatively few viewers (1,000 to 2,500 views). LVCT Health has a Facebook page, with articles, pictures, and event updates, yet relatively few links to videos. Further consideration could be given to developing a comprehensive program developing and promoting videos on HIV/AIDS in KSL that could be accessed on YouTube or on a government or NGO website. Accessible video materials in KSL can support the health literacy of Deaf Kenyans.

An explosive growth of mobile phones in Kenya has also opened up possibilities for mHealth as a means to increase mobility and address the enduring problems of education, communication, stigma, privacy, and treatment for Deaf Kenyans. In 2015, mobile penetration reached 83 percent of the population, and 58 percent of the units sold that year were smartphones; 99 percent of the owners of smartphones accessed the Internet via mobile technology (Zab 2015). In 2011, the World Health Organization (WHO)—with the assistance of experts in 114 countries—issued a landmark report, *mHealth: New Horizons for Health through Mobile Technologies.* The report noted that the expansion of mobile phone networks in low- and middle-income lands (like Kenya) often surpassed other national infrastructures, such as paved roads and electricity, as well as fixed Internet systems (WHO 2011). Yet health sectors have generally been slow to capitalize on mobile technology. WHO issued a call for a coordinated worldwide movement for the development and evaluation of mHealth to improve access to health information, records, and monitoring of chronic conditions, arguing that "mHealth can revolutionize health outcomes, providing virtually anyone with a mobile phone with medical expertise and knowledge in real time. This is a boon particularly to those marginalized or living in remote areas, who would otherwise not have access to this information or care" (WHO 2011: 77).

While a comprehensive mHealth strategy for Deaf Kenyans has not yet been developed, specific applications of mobile technology to HIV/AIDS care have been introduced into Kenya for other groups. For example, shortly after the WHO report, the CDC Foundation (n.d.) and mHealth Kenya developed innovative mobile treatment and monitoring systems for health workers potentially exposed to HIV infections, and for infants born to mothers with HIV. Moreover, Horvath et al. (2012), in a meta-analysis, found that mobile text messaging improved medication adherence to ARV therapy. This has implications for HIV+ Deaf Kenyans in rural areas.

Wildermuth (2013: 55) notes the special potential of information and communication technology (ICT) in Kenya: "Contemporarily, Kenya, and in specific Nairobi, is the site of an innovative environment for the cooperation between social change agents and IT experts around issues of e-citizenship, e-democracy and digital empowerment." Along the same lines, "Kenya has become a popular location for the design and implementation of mediated spaces for civic engagement and of participatory communication initiatives for social change" (Wildermuth 2013: 73). Furthermore, "Nairobi, in particular, has blossomed as an African hub for the design and development of mobile phone- and Web-based applications for social change" (Wildermuth 2013: 58). ICT has potential to advance the communication strategies of civil society organizations like LVCT Health. Nevertheless, that potential is limited by economic barriers to access ICT and the need for funding and programs to make technology widely available to all strata of Kenyan society. Wildermuth's (2013) conception of "digital empowerment" will be critical in making Deaf Kenyans full citizens in the age of HIV/AIDS.

A cautionary note is required. Despite its great promise, mHealth is not a magic bullet for all forms of immobility. Mobile technology is just that, a technology, not a substitute for a well-conceived and articulated health program. This is particularly true for Deaf Kenyan PLWHA in rural areas, especially if they are not literate, since sending text message reminders for ARV treatment may be less effective than it would be with other populations and may need to be used in conjunction with existing peer-led mobile VCT outreach strategies. At best, it can serve as a complementary strategy for a program such as that of LVCT Health for Deaf Kenyans. According to a summary of African mobile health initiatives, "creating useful mHealth applications isn't about throwing up a website that is useful for government organizations; it's about understanding needs on the ground" ("Quick Rundown" 2012). Toward that end, developers of mHealth applications would be wise to follow LVCT Health's groundbreaking community and peer-based approach, involving those to be served in developing countries and directing programs to meet their own health needs.

Lessons Learned

LVCT Health continues to focus on serving people with disabilities, although formal Deaf VCT services were discontinued in 2011 due to lack of funds. The experience of LVCT Health underscores the importance of participatory communication so that Deaf Kenyans are positioned to provide peer-based, peer-led, and accessible services to their community (Freire 2000). A further step in this regard would be to strive to overcome stigma so that greater numbers of openly HIV+ Deaf Kenyans could join the ranks of service providers. Moreover, progress in addressing the needs of the Deaf in regard to HIV/AIDS must be linked to the broader principles of social change communication (SCC) in which communities control the channels for their own advancement. That advancement needs to be linked to improvement in both economic conditions and access to resources, including communication technology. As Chandwani and Gopal (2010: 23) write,

> Understanding the dynamics of HIV transmission can't be separated from an understanding of the broader context of poverty, inequality and social exclusion which create conditions where unsafe behavior flourishes. Social change communication can tackle structural drivers of the HIV epidemic, with a particular focus on the drivers of gender inequality, stigma and discrimination, and human rights violations. Social change communication is bound to emerge as the vaccine and panacea for HIV and AIDS.

The impact of mHealth innovations will depend on whether Deaf Kenyans have the mobility to control and use its tools in accordance with the principles of SCC. The mission of an organization such as LVCT Health might be more fully realized by selectively exploiting the potential of mHealth. To return to Susan Sontag's metaphor, a smartphone could serve as a Deaf Kenyan's passport for medical citizenship in facing the challenge of HIV/AIDS.

Alina Engelman, DrPH, MPH, is an assistant professor of health sciences at California State University, East Bay, and on the Community Health Commission for the City of Berkeley. She is an affiliated researcher at University of California, Berkeley, with a focus on health initiatives for underserved populations. As part of her graduate studies in global health at Yale University, she received the Lindsey Fellowship for Research in Africa (Kenya) from the Yale University Center for International and Area Studies. Her interests include health disparities, health literacy, program evaluation, and emergency preparedness for at-risk populations.

NOTES

1. The uppercase "Deaf" is used to indicate a cultural orientation denoting membership in a linguistic minority group, while the lowercase "deaf" refers to deafness as purely a medical condition. In this chapter, the term is capitalized to honor how Deaf Kenyans themselves have chosen to identify their community. The author recognizes that the capitalization of "Deaf" originated from American scholarship and can carry a different meaning in other contexts (Senghas and Monaghan 2002; LeMaster 2003; Woodward 1972).
2. The study provided the basis for the author's MPH thesis (Engelman 2007).
3. "Anne" is a pseudonym, used to protect her privacy and confidentiality.
4. "Jane" is a pseudonym, used to protect her privacy and confidentiality.

REFERENCES

Adoyo, Peter O. 2007. "Educating Deaf Children in an Inclusive Setting in Kenya: Challenges and Considerations." *Electronic Journal for Inclusive Education* 2(2): 1–13.

Biggs, Nalini Asha. 2013. "HIV/AIDS Education in Kenyan Schools for the Deaf." Extended Abstract. MLitt thesis. Oxford, UK: University of Oxford. Retrieved 16 March 2018 from https://sites.google.com/site/naliniasha/research/current-research-hiv-aids-education-in-kenyan-schools-for-the-deaf.

Boal, A. 2000. *Theater of the Oppressed.* London: Pluto Press.

Büscher, Monika, and John Urry. 2009. "Mobile Methods and the Empirical." *European Journal of Social Theory* 12(1): 99–116.Cardey, Sarah, Chris Garforth, Eliza Govender, and Lauren Dyll-Myklebust. 2013. "Entertainment Education Theory and Practice in HIV/AIDS Communication: A South Africa/United Kingdom Comparison." *Critical Arts* 27(3): 288–310.

CDC Foundation. n.d. "Mobile Health: How Phones Are Reshaping Healthcare in Africa." Retrieved 29 April 2016 from http://www.cdcfoundation.org/content/mobile-health-how-phones-are-reshaping-healthcare-africa.

Chandwani, Haresh, and Rajesh Gopal. 2010. "Social Change Communication: Need of the Hour for the Prevention of HIV/AIDS." *Journal of Clinical Medicine Research* 2(1): 23–26.

D'Andrea, Anthony, Luigina Ciolfi, and Breda Gray. 2011. "Methodological Challenges and Innovations in Mobilities Research." *Mobilities* 6(2): 149–60.

Engelman, Alina. 2006. "A Qualitative Evaluation of Deaf VCT Services in Kenya: Policy Recommendations for Community-Based Capacity Building." Policy Report. Kenya: Liverpool VCT (LVCT Health).

———. 2007. "Deaf Kenyans At-Risk for HIV/AIDS: A Situational Assessment of Need." MPH thesis. New Haven, CT: Yale University.

Freire, Paulo. 2000. *Pedagogy of the Oppressed.* New York: Continuum.

Friedner, Michele. 2014. "Deaf Capital: An Exploration of the Relationship between Stigma and Value in Deaf Multilevel Marketing Participation in Urban India." *Medical Anthropology Quarterly* 28(4): 502–18.

Gallaudet University. "Kenya." *Office of Research Support and International Affairs.* Retrieved 16 March 2018 from http://www.gallaudet.edu/research-support-and-international-affairs/international-affairs/world-deaf-information-resource/deaf-orgs/local-orgs/kenya.

Groce, Nora. 2006. "HIV/AIDS and Disability: A Pilot Survey of HIV/AIDS Knowledge among a Deaf Population in Swaziland," *International Journal of Rehabilitation Research* 29(4): 319–24.

Hatar, A., 2005. "Are We Answering the Right Questions? Challenges for Participatory Development Communication among the Barbaig in Northern Tanzania." *Tanzanian Journal of Development Studies*, 6(1): 147–163.

Hivos. 2014. "Documentation of Best Practices in Programming with Key Populations in the Context of HIV/AIDS in Kenya." Report presented to LVCT Health. Retrieved 13

July 2016 from https://www.hivos.nl/assets/2015/10/LVCT-Best-Practices-Documentantion-Report-FINAL-August.pdf.

Horvath, Tara, Hana Azman, Gail E. Kennedy, and George W. Rutherford. 2012. "Mobile Phone Text Messaging for Promoting Adherence to Antiretroviral Therapy in Patients with HIV Infection." *Cochrane Database of Systematic Reviews,* 3: CD009756. doi:10.1002/14651858.CD009756.

LeMaster, Barbara. 2003. "School Language and Shifts in Irish Deaf Identity." In *Many Ways to Be Deaf: International Variation in Deaf Communities,* ed. Leila Monaghan, Constanze, Schmaling, Karen Nakamura, and Graham Turner, 153–72. Washington, DC: Gallaudet University Press.

LVCT Health. 2014. *Strategy 2014–2017.* Nairobi, Kenya: LVCT Head Office.

———. 2016a. "Strategy 2014-2017." Retrieved 16 March 2018 from lvcthealth.org/wp-content/uploads/2017/09/strategy-2014-2017-strategy.pdf.

———. 2016b. "Populations We Serve." Retrieved 16 March 2018 from http://lvcthealth.org/what-we-do/populations-we-serve/.

———. 2016c. "Training Institute." Retrieved 16 March 2018 from http://www.lvcthealth.org/training-institute.

Macharia, Ken. 2015. "70 Percent of Kenyans Now Have Access to the Internet." *Capital Business,* 4 August. Retrieved 13 July 2016 from http://www.capitalfm.co.ke/business/2015/08/70-percent-of-kenyans-now-have-access-to-the-internet.

Manyozo, Linje. 2013. "Communication for Development in Sub-Saharan Africa: From Orientalism to NGOification." In *Speaking Up and Talking Back? Media, Empowerment, and Civic Engagement among East and Southern African Youth,* ed. Thomas Tufte, Norbert Wildermuth, Sofie Anne Hansen-Skovmoes, and Winnie Mitullah, 37–52. Gothenburg: International Clearinghouse on Children, Youth, and Media.

Opiyo, W., L. Muruka, and A. Engelman. 2006. "Interviews with Job Candidates at Coast Deaf VCT." Formal unpublished document. Kenya.

"Quick Rundown of African Mobile Health Initiatives." 2012. *Africa: Tracking Internet Progress,* 2 December. Retrieved on13 July 2016 from http://www.oafrica.com/education/quick-rundown-of-african-mobile-health-initiatives/.

Salazar, Noel, and Alan Smart. 2011. "Anthropological Takes on (Im)mobility." *Identities: Global Studies in Culture and Power* 18(6): i–ix.

Schenker, Inon I. 2005. "HIV/AIDS Literacy: An Essential Component in Education for All." Paper commissioned for the *EFA Global Monitoring Report 2006: Literacy for Life.* UNESCO. Retrieved 16 March 2018 from http://unesdoc.unesco.org/images/0014/001461/146182e.pdf.

Senghas, Richard J., and Monaghan, Leila. 2002. "Signs of Their Times: Deaf Communities and the Culture of Language." *Annual Review of Anthropology* 31: 69–97.

Shackleton, Joanna. 2009. "Exploring Perceptions of Deaf Persons for Recommendations towards Effective HIV/AIDS Programming in Nairobi." *Journal of Human Development, Disability, and Social Change* 18(2): 59–76.

Sheller, Meghan. 2006. "View of Young People in Kisumu District on HIV/AIDS and Marriage." MA thesis. Cedar Falls, IA: University of Northern Iowa.

Sontag, Susan. 1970. *Illness as Metaphor.* New York: Farrar, Straus and Giroux.

Taegtmeyer, M., A. Hightower, W. Opiyo, L. Mwachiro, K. Henderson, P. Angala, C. Ngare, and E. Marum. 2009. "A Peer-Led HIV Counseling and Testing Programme for the Deaf in Kenya." *Journal of Disability and Rehabilitation* 31(6): 508–14.

Ubido J., J. Huntington, and D. Warburton. 2002. "Inequalities in Access to Healthcare Faced by Women Who Are Deaf." *Health and Social Care in the Community* 10(4): 247–53.

WHO (World Health Organization). 2011. *mHealth: New Horizons for Health through Mobile Technologies.* Global Observatory for eHealth Series, Vol. 3. Geneva: WHO.

Wildermuth, Norbert. 2013. "Information and Communication Technology-Facilitated E-citizenship, E-democracy and Digital Empowerment in Kenya: The Opportunities and Constraints of Community-Based Initiatives." In *Speaking Up and Talking Back? Media, Empowerment, and Civic Engagement among East and Southern African Youth,* ed. Thomas Tufte, Norbert Wildermuth, Sofie Anne Hansen-Skovmoes, and Winnie Mitullah, 11–18. Gothenburg: International Clearinghouse on Children, Youth, and Media.

Wohlfeiler, Dan. 2002. "Community Organizing and Community Building among Gay and Bisexual Men." In *Community Organizing and Community Building for Health,* ed. Meredith Minkler, 230–243. New Brunswick, NJ: Rutgers University Press.

Woodward, J. C. 1972. "Implications for Sociolinguistic Research among the Deaf." *Sign Language Studies* 1(1): 1–7.

World Bank. 2014. "Access to Electricity (% of Population)." Sustainable Energy for All (SE4ALL) database. Retrieved on 11 December 2017 from https://data.worldbank.org/indicator/EG.ELC.ACCS.ZS.

———. 2016. "Rural Population (% of Total Population)." Retrieved 25 April 2016 from http://data.worldbank.org/indicator/SP.RUR.TOTL.ZS.

Zab, Sofia. 2015. "Whitepaper: The Growth of the Smartphone Market in Kenya." *Jumia,* 2 June. Retrieved on 13 July 2016 from https://www.jumia.co.ke/blog/whitepaper-the-growth-of-the-smartphone-market-in-kenya.

CHAPTER
8

Service-Learning Research Projects to Enhance the Information Accompanying Commonly Dispensed Medicines on the Phelophepa Healthcare Trains

Sunitha C. Srinivas and Sharli A. Paphitis

Public health in developing countries requires health promotion strategies that use innovative methods of delivery in order for desired levels of up-take to be achieved—specifically, in the delivery of services to rural, hard-to-reach populations whose mobility is limited in various ways. Physical access to healthcare facilities has implications for population health, but it has been notoriously difficult to assess and determine physical access to healthcare in developing countries, where an array of geographic, sociodemographic, behavioral, and societal factors affect the utilization of facilities (Tanser, Gijsbertsen, and Herbst 2006). The geographic accessibility of healthcare facilities and services has been shown to impact not only the utilization of these facilities and services, but, consequently, specific health outcomes such as maternal and infant mortality, adverse pregnancy outcomes, contraceptive use, immunizations, and adherence to tuberculosis and HIV/AIDS treatment regimens (McLaren, Ardington, and Leibbrandt 2013; Tanser et al. 2006). While geographical constraints play an important role in the physical mobility of patients, access to healthcare is embedded in a network of intersecting mobilities across physical, epistemic, and cultural divides and distances (Salazar, Elliot, and Norum 2017). In South Africa, the intimate links between physical mobility and other forms of mobility (such as mobility within socioeconomic systems or within the epistemic realm of health literacy) highlight the important ways in which, in the context of access to healthcare, "geographical movement is always invested with social meaning" (Salazar et al. 2017: 6).

In the South African context, there is inadequate coverage of the basic healthcare needs of the poorer majority of the population who live in remote and rural areas (Truter 2010, 2013). While progress has been made in South Africa since the end of apartheid, disparities in access to healthcare remain a central concern in breaking cycles of entrenched poverty and inequality. Despite increased healthcare facilities in remote rural areas, the most vulnerable members of society face barriers—such as affordability and travel time—that are significant and remain disparate along racial and gender lines (McLaren et al. 2013). Nationally, it is estimated that 17 percent of South Africans spend over one hour traveling to access public healthcare facilities (of the rural population, 31 percent report travel times of more than one hour), with 49 percent of the population walking to access those facilities (Tanser et al. 2006). Maldistribution of finances, resources, and workers between rural and urban areas (as well as between private and public sectors) compromises health coverage for South Africa's large, vulnerable, and underserved rural population. While in urban provinces (Gauteng and Western Cape) 1,234 professional nurses were produced in 2014, the three much larger rural provinces of Limpopo, North West, and Northern Cape produced only 50, and in 2010 there were 100,000 reported public sector vacancies (Rispel 2016). Disparities in annual healthcare expenditure per capita are also vast: US$1,500 (R 12,000) in the private sector, which serves approximately 16 percent of the population, predominantly in urban areas; and US$150 (R 1,200) in the public sector, serving 84 percent of the population, the majority of whom live in rural areas. All this is indicative of the human and material resources that would be required to bring about equity for individuals receiving care under these distinct systems and thus to bridge the divide between two distinct spaces of healthcare (Benatar 2013).

South Africans make up 17 percent of the global population with HIV/AIDS, and South Africa is reported to have one of the highest incidences of tuberculosis worldwide, following only India and China (Benatar 2013; WHO 2014). Although South Africa boasts the largest global antiretroviral (ARV) treatment program, only 40 percent of eligible South Africans are receiving treatment, due to the influence of adverse social forces, and of those on ARV treatment only 40 percent are able to reach WHO standards for optimum adherence (Benatar 2013; Kagee et al. 2011; Van Dyk 2011). Structural as well as socioeconomic and cultural barriers have been widely identified to be the primary factors affecting patient nonadherence: studies have specifically identified factors such as lack of transport, food scarcity, lack of social support, inadequate medical care and mental health care services, and generalized low health literacy, as well as a specific lack of knowledge and understanding of medication and treatment regimens, stigma, and relationship with healthcare workers (Kagee et al. 2011; Naidoo et al. 2013; Van Dyk 2011). Similarly, adverse social and cultural forces are seen to impact the increased prevalence of noncommunicable diseases, as well as adherence to treatment regimens or preventive measures for these diseases, across South Africa (where drug adherence for patients taking chronic medication is between 40 and 50 percent).

All of these health issues could be addressed through increased health literacy, improved relationships with healthcare workers, and effective, culturally relevant health promotion. This paints an overarching picture in which solutions to health pandemics, which are rooted in sociocultural and political conditions, seem unlikely to be addressed solely through biomedical interventions (Benatar 2013; Van Dyk 2011). From the perspective of the "new mobilities paradigm" (Sheller and Urry 2006), for the predominantly rural, hard-to-reach population in South Africa, public health can be neither understood nor addressed on the basis of systems of physical or geographical mobility alone. Healthcare must be understood in terms of movement between epistemic spaces of health literacy, as well as between healthcare providers and patients in spaces of cultural divide and difference.

Health literacy, most basically, is the term used to indicate an individual's ability to access, understand, and use information promoting their health and well-being. Low levels of health literacy are commonly noted among the elderly and those with low educational attainment (Wong 2012). Written materials can be provided to increase patients' ability to make informed decisions about their healthcare and to reinforce the need for positive behavioral changes. Such materials offer a number of benefits, including message consistency, reusability, portability, and self-paced learning. As most patients frequently forget the verbal information that their healthcare practitioner provides, written materials have the added benefit of aiding in recall and reinforcing such information. However, these advantages are valuable only to patients who can read and understand the materials provided. Poor health outcomes can be attributed to low levels of health literacy (Sheridan et al. 2011). For patients, low health literacy results in an inability to read, interpret, and follow instructions—hence, they are unlikely to understand medication information, because they tend to struggle with interpreting medication labels, auxiliary labels, directions for use, and written and verbal information (Wali and Grindrod 2016). As a result, patients with low literacy skills tend to use more health services than those with higher literacy levels (Center on an Aging Society 2004).

Cognitive and literacy demands on patients are becoming more rigorous than ever with the growing complexities of modern healthcare systems. "Medication literacy" is a crucial component of the broader concept of "health literacy," where oral and written information are essential to ensuring that patients use medications safely and effectively (Raynor 2013). Globally, research demonstrates that increasing rates of health literacy, including medication literacy, could potentially lead to advances in informed decision making by patients, a reduction of health risks, increases in prevention and wellness, improved quality of life, and better navigation of the health system and patient safety and care (Bann et al. 2012). Particularly within contexts such as these, innovative strategies to improve public health mobility must be employed; they can overcome a myriad of socioeconomic, cultural, and environmental challenges, such as a critical lack of manpower, lack of accessible and affordable healthcare, low levels of health literacy, and the negative attitudes of healthcare professionals toward treating the poor or underserved.

In this chapter, we discuss intersecting interventions in which unique technologies are being mobilized to improve public health and health promotion in South Africa along these fault lines, from large-scale, country-wide interventions to small-scale interactions between healthcare students and their local communities. Within this chapter, the concepts of mobility, constraint, and access play a central role: movement and stasis between or within spaces in the physical, epistemic, and cultural realms can be seen as a barrier or a bridge to accessibility in public health. While much attention is currently being given to the potential benefit of modern or new technologies, such as cellular phones, in improving access to public health, our chapter highlights that what constitutes effective "new" technologies in the development context may instead involve revitalizing old infrastructure and well-known machinery, as in the case of the Phelophepa Trains, to increase affordability of and access to primary healthcare for rural, hard-to-reach populations. Additionally, returning to early modes of communication, such as pictographic representations on patient information leaflets, to bridge the gap between linguistic, cultural, and educational divides in health literacy is a key concept in our chapter. Common to the interventions discussed in this chapter is the notion that improved access to healthcare—in physical, epistemic, and ontological terms—can only be achieved through navigating a variety of cultural contestations surrounding access for diverse South African populations. While the relationship between healthcare workers and patients is at the heart of many of these contestations, the interventions discussed here show ways in which a new generation of healthcare workers are learning to move effectively within the cultural context of health promotion in post-apartheid South Africa.

The Phelophepa Trains

One successful approach to providing primary healthcare services to hard-to-reach populations has been the utilization of mobile clinics, which can provide cost-effective and easily accessible points of contact to healthcare (Bassett et al. 2014; Hill et al. 2012; Maheswaran et al. 2012; Oriol et al. 2009; Truter 2010; Vos, Borgdorff, and Kachidza 1990). The Phelophepa Train(s) is one such mobile healthcare initiative. It has been operational in South Africa since 1994 and now comprises two 16-coach Trains carrying modern medical equipment and staff (Truter 2013). "Phelophepa" (pay-lo-pe-pa) is a word meaning "good clean health" in a combination of two local South African languages, Tswana and Sotho, and the Phelophepa Trains run on over 9,320 miles (15,000 km) of railway tracks, enabling the provision of primary healthcare services and health education in remote and rural areas that have limited access to healthcare facilities (Hansraj 2009; Jacobs 2004; Jacobs, MacKenzie, and Botma 2013; Truter 2013). The Trains travel to designated stations in eight provinces across South Africa according to an annual roster, where they remain stationed for one to two weeks (Bhayat et al. 2011). The Trains offer holistic services to communities in the remote surrounding areas in the primary healthcare fields of optometry, nursing, dentistry, pharmacy, and psychology (Jacobs et al. 2013; Hansraj 2009; Bhayat et al. 2011). More than a decade after the initiative's inception in 1994, the Trains have reached over 23.5 million people through onboard services and training programs; in 2008 alone, a total of 26,970 prescriptions were issued from the onboard pharmacy facility (Hansraj 2009; Truter 2013; American Friends of the Phelophepa Train 2015). The most common conditions treated by healthcare workers on the

Train are ear infections, skin infections, chest infections, urinary tract infections, sexually transmitted diseases, diarrhea, dental caries, periodontitis, musculoskeletal conditions, minor eye diseases, and genitourinary system conditions (Truter 2010, 2013). Medications are primarily prescribed by nurses and dispensed by the pharmacists on board the Train, with medications from the Primary Healthcare Essential Drug List being dispensed (Truter 2010).

The South African Phelophepa primary healthcare Train is a unique initiative in the mobile healthcare arena for two reasons, beyond it being the first and only primary healthcare Train in the world (Truter 2010, 2013). First, the initiative serves not only as a mobile healthcare delivery program, but also as a unique training site for students enrolled in health-related disciplines at higher education institutions. Second, the initiative takes a holistic approach to healthcare delivery, including health promotion and educational activities, while also adopting a community-centered approach to primary healthcare delivery. This enables the mobile Train to respond to issues of physical accessibility as well as to a host of interrelated issues of cultural and epistemic accessibility.

Funding for Phelophepa comes from both the public and private sectors; the initiative has a close partnership with the South African government, particularly the Departments of Health and Social Development, as well as higher education institutions across South Africa (Bhayat et al. 2011). Annually, an average of 895 international exchange students as well as South African students, in their final year of study or at a postgraduate level in health-related disciplines at partner higher education institutions, work as volunteers in rotation aboard the Train as part of their study programs to gain practical experience in a clinical environment (Bayat et al. 2011; Hansraj 2009; Jacobs et al. 2013; Jacobs 2004; Truter 2013). Numerous studies on the experiences of students working and learning aboard the Trains have reported that the Trains provide students with the opportunity to develop their professional skills (including clinical and diagnostic skills and in patient care) through hands-on experience in a unique setting where they are afforded the opportunity to make judgments with relative independence and to work collaboratively in a multidisciplinary healthcare environment (Hansraj 2009; Jacobs et al. 2013; Truter 2013).

Importantly, Phelophepa is a community-centered initiative, and community nurses head up reconnaissance teams that visit sites serviced by the Trains up to twelve weeks before the Trains arrive, to establish the healthcare needs and concerns in local contexts (Jacobs 2004). The initiative also intentionally adopts an approach that focuses on health promotion, health education, and preventive medication through the inclusion of an onboard "Edu-Clinic," where education initiatives aimed at disseminating information to the broader surrounding communities are run (Jacobs et al. 2013; Jacobs 2004; Koodibetse 2015). Given that students working on the Trains gain hands-on experience in a community setting, research has shown that the students show improved communication and interpersonal skills, moral growth, and an increased awareness of both the cultural diversity of the South African context and the public health needs in community (particularly rural) settings (Bhayat et al. 2011; Hansraj 2009; Jacobs et al. 2013; Truter 2013).

Cultural exposure and the opportunity to work closely with patients on the Train allows students to gain a deeper understanding of South African culture more generally, but in particular, it allows students to come to understand how to work with a diverse group of patients by giving the students insight into and sensitivity toward patient problems, needs, and cultural backgrounds. In providing this kind of training for the next generation of healthcare professionals in South Africa, the Phelophepa initiative takes a critical step toward addressing one of the most significant barriers to healthcare delivery to rural, hard-to-reach populations: the negative attitudes of healthcare professionals toward treating the poor or underserved.

While the Train is perceived to be a beneficial and outstanding community-centered site for clinical training for students in health-related disciplines, providing students with learning opportunities beyond mere clinical or discipline-specific knowledge and skill acquisition, students have reported significant difficulties in attempting to provide effective healthcare delivery onboard the Trains (Hansraj 2009; Jacobs et al. 2013; Truter 2013). Students and staff aboard Phelophepa are often expected to work exceedingly long hours, because the Train remains in an area for only a short period of time and patients stay at the station until they have been attended to. This may present a significant barrier to care, given that long-term illnesses cannot be monitored and follow-up consultations cannot be scheduled (Bhayat et al. 2011; Hansraj 2009; Jacobs 2004; Truter 2013).

Health Literacy and Medicines Information Leaflets

Currently, five pharmacy faculties from South African higher education institutions—Nelson Mandela Metropolitan University, University of Kwa-zulu-Natal, the University of Witwatersrand, the University of Limpopo, and Rhodes University—partner with the Phelophepa initiative, with each institution sending fourteen students to work on the Trains annually. The pharmacy aboard the Train is staffed by two final-year students from the partner higher education institutions under the supervision of two qualified pharmacists and a translator. The need for a translator is significant in a hetroglossic society such as South Africa (with eleven official languages, forty-four living languages, and a large immigrant and refugee population). Medical interactions typically take place in English, resulting in 80 percent of these interactions occurring across language barriers, making language and culture often more of a barrier to effective healthcare than socioeconomic issues in South Africa (Benjamin et al. 2016; Hagan et al. 2013). In the Phelophepa pharmacy, the role of the translator in interpreting and translating instructions for the medication dispensed is critical for the rational use of medication and subsequent patient adherence. This role is particularly important on the Trains that serve a primarily low-literate population, who rely on pharmacist's verbal communication and instructions for the rational use of prescribed medications rather than the enclosed patient information leaflets that typically accompany the drugs dispensed. Barriers to effective patient care reported by students on the Phelophepa Trains working through translators are significant and require careful consideration (by staff at universities who partner with the Phelophepa initiative) for addressing not only primary healthcare in the form of health literacy, but the training of healthcare professionals to effectively communicate with a diverse population without exhibiting biases or prejudice.

Health literacy first appeared as a concept for serious study in academic peer-reviewed literature in the early 1990s, but by 2011 there were 569 peer-reviewed publications on the topic (Pleasant 2013). It is increasingly recognized as a distinct form of literacy, with important repercussions for socioeconomic and health development. Typically, health literacy is understood to refer to a set of skills or capacities exhibited by individuals that allow them to effectively take part in healthcare environments and activities, including basic literacy and numeracy skills in order to read and understand prescriptions, patient information and appointment records, and essential health materials (Baker 2006). A recent systematic review of the existing health literacy literature by Sørensen et al. (2015: 1053) sets out an integrated definition of health literacy that describes what it means to effectively take part in healthcare environments: "the knowledge, motivation and competences to access, understand, appraise and apply health information in order to make judgments and take decisions in everyday life concerning health care, disease prevention and health promotion to maintain or improve quality of life throughout the course of life." Such a definition sees health literacy as, in part, relational as well as dynamic, relating both to the individual and the healthcare system in which they are operating (Baker 2006). Health knowledge also plays an important part in this definition and can be understood to comprise distinct realms that together contribute to health literacy: oral literacy, print literacy, numeracy, and conceptual and cultural knowledge (Baker 2006). Again, there is an important interplay here between the individual and the healthcare system in which they operate, since the measurement of a person's health-related print and oral literacy depends on their health-related reading fluency (i.e., vocabulary) and the complexity of the texts or oral communications they encounter in their healthcare environment (Baker 2006).

Unfortunately, the concept of health literacy is conspicuously absent from South Africa's governmental health policies (Pleasant 2013). This is particularly concerning given that access to both education and healthcare services is inadequate for a high proportion of the South African population. The National Drug Policy for South Africa, however, incorporates a section on rational use of medicines that stipulates that medicine-related literature be understandable by the public. The policy highlights the importance of providing objective, validated, and practical information on use of medicines appropriate to the literacy levels of the population. The crucial role of pharmacists in conveying medicines information to the public is also reiterated in the policy (National Department of Health 1996).

While health literacy as nomenclature may be absent, policy documents indicate that the South African government is shifting toward the need for increased efforts to facilitate understanding by patients (Pleasant 2013). Similarly, South Africa's National Department of Health stipulates in its Policy on Language Services (National Department of Health 2011) that providers of medicines are responsible for ensuring that product information and inset documentation are made available in at least two of the nation's eleven official languages. However, English and Afrikaans are the languages predominantly used for medicines information leaflets (MILs), which excludes the majority of the underserved population, especially those in rural areas, for whom neither English nor Afrikaans is spoken either as a first or a second language. While international policy seems to be increasingly taking into account countries with low health literacy rates and widespread illiteracy, such as South Africa, MILs that accompany medication are often not only misunderstood, but not understood at all. Practical solutions to achieving greater health literacy with regards to MILs have therefore not come from policy directives.

Research conducted with Rhodes University Pharmacy faculty points to an innovative solution to meeting the health literacy needs of underserved South African populations in the form of culturally and contextually relevant pictograms, which can be used to supplement MILs. While patients' inability to understand MILs that accompany medicines is thought to be a major factor in the lack of rational medicine use (as well as contributing to nonadherence), the introduction of pictograms to supplement written MILs has been found to have a positive impact on both understanding and adherence in patients with low health literacy (Dowse and Ehlers 2001, 2005).

This has been shown to be the case specifically when the pictograms are culturally sensitive or contextually relevant to the designated population (Dowse and Ehlers 2001).

Service-Learning Research Projects in Health Literacy

Service-learning health research projects conducted by South African universities within local contexts not only provide students with opportunities to engage with diverse and complex cultural communities in a practical way, but also ensure that they achieve the critical cross-field outcomes (CCFOs) stipulated by the South African Qualifications Authority in the National Qualifications Framework and Curriculum Development (SAQA 2000). These CCFOs form part of the institutional policies at Rhodes University. Graduates are expected to gain the following critical abilities: to identify and solve problems, to work in a team, to organize and manage themselves, to use science and technology, to recognize problem-solving contexts, to reflect on and explore effective learning strategies, to participate as a responsible citizen, to be culturally and aesthetically sensitive, and to explore education and career opportunities. Service-learning activities such as these are aimed at producing graduates who will go on to be well-rounded citizens and professionals, capable of navigating the cultural complexities and divides faced in South Africa, particularly within the healthcare industry.

It is with these CCFOs in mind that this service-learning course was designed, in which students would be actively involved in the development and testing of pictographic MILs for medications distributed on the Phelophepa Trains. This course aimed to familiarize students with the intrinsically social and cultural nature of health literacy by allowing them to develop culturally and contextually relevant pictographic MILs and to gain hands-on experience in interacting with patients from the designated population group (those with both low literacy and low health literacy rates) in the process of testing the pictographic MILs. Through the students' research projects, pictographic MILs have been developed for use by students and pharmacists working on the Phelophepa Train. Plans for distribution of MILs on the Trains, and for further field testing and feedback from end users, are currently being discussed.

Methods

Third-year pharmacy students worked in teams to conduct service-learning research projects. Each team was provided an assessment grid for each step of the research process that would be used to mark their final projects.

The final projects included: forming a team and drafting a social norms contract, a research proposal, three drafts of MILs, and a final research report. Groups were guided through the process of delegating the various tasks among themselves and assigning tasks and responsibilities according to each member's personal aptitude and capabilities. While this exercise was useful logistically, it also addressed a key CCFO: problem solving. Each group attended a workshop on ethics and research, and another on the design of MILs.

During the service-learning program, the third-year pharmacy students were supervised over a period of two years. Students were divided into groups of five, and each group was assigned one of the thirteen most important medications specifically distributed by the Phelophepa Trains (as identified by Phelophepa staff): Allergex (chlorphenamine); amoxicillin; aspirin; benzyl benzoate lotion; ciprofloxacin; Codoxol (paracetamol, codeine, caffeine, doxylamine); cyclizine; doxycycline; erythromycin; ibuprofen; metronidazole; Rehidrat (an oral rehydration salt formulation in a sachet); and Sinuend (paracetamol, ephedrine hydrochloride, caffeine, chlorphenamine maleate (synchlorpheniramine). Each student group was assigned a medication from this list and tasked with designing a culturally and context-specific pictographic MIL for their assigned medication. The task of designing their MILs involved an iterative process of testing pictographic MILs for cultural appropriateness, readability, and comprehension with a sample population with both low literacy and low health literacy rates.

Students developed and tested their pictographic MILs through a rigorous consultation and drafting process with course coordinators (after having submitted research proposals for ethical clearance) and then subsequently with the sample population of community participants. The pictographic MILs and research reports developed by students supervised in the first year of the service-learning program formed the foundation for continued development in the second year of the program, ensuring that the service-learning projects underwent extensive and rigorous testing before being implemented for field testing by staff of the Phelophepa Trains, which is the next stage of the program.

Results

After initial feedback by the research coordinator on the first draft of the pictographic MILs, students consulted representative sample groups comprised of individuals with both low literacy and low health literacy for the production of a second (pilot testing) and third draft, finally reformulating their pictographic MILs based on qualitative feedback from their community participants (see Figures 8.1, 8.2, and 8.3 for examples of pictographic MILs developed by students within the service-learning program).

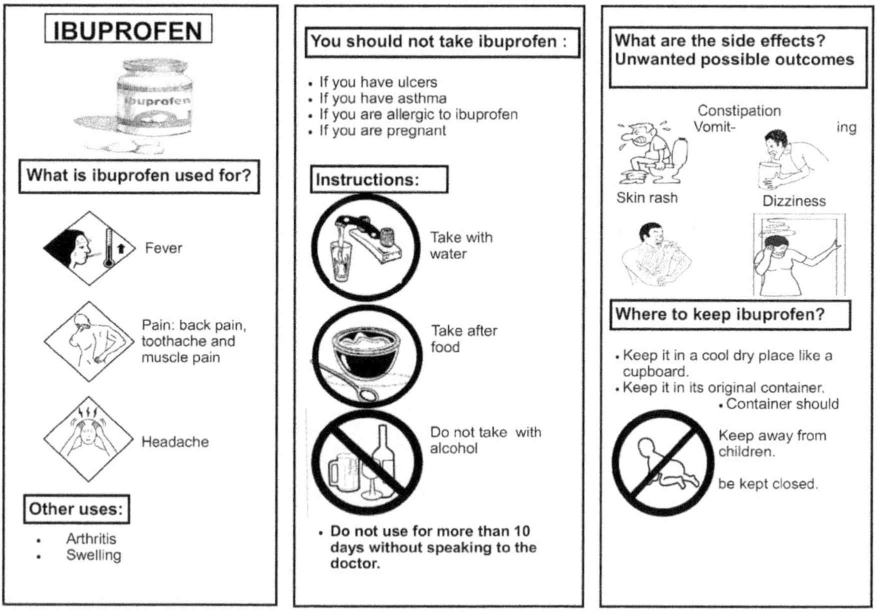

Figure 8.1 Ibuprofen pictographic MIL developed by third-year pharmacy students. Figure by the authors.

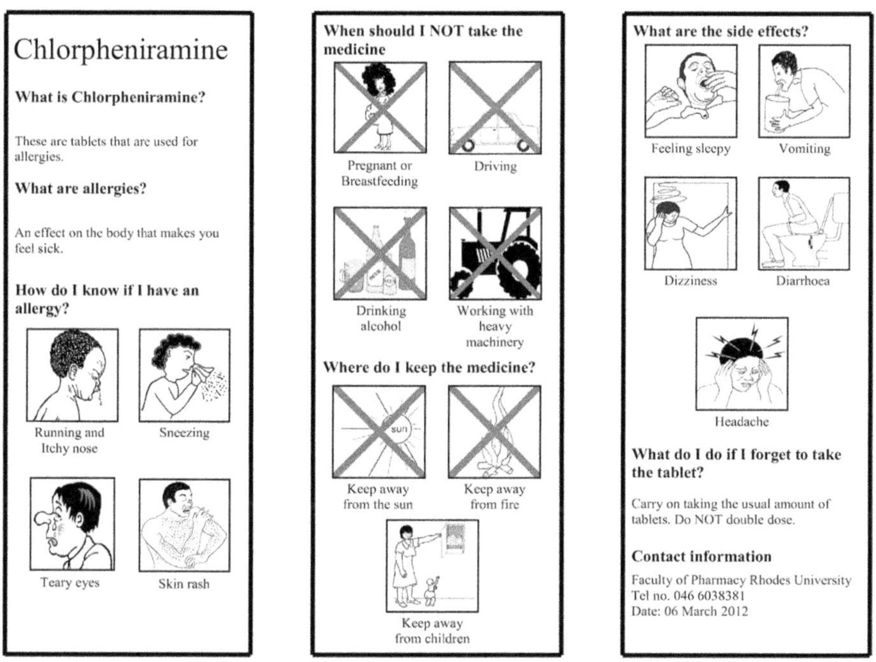

Figure 8.2 Chlorpheniramine pictographic MIL developed by third-year pharmacy students. Figure by the authors.

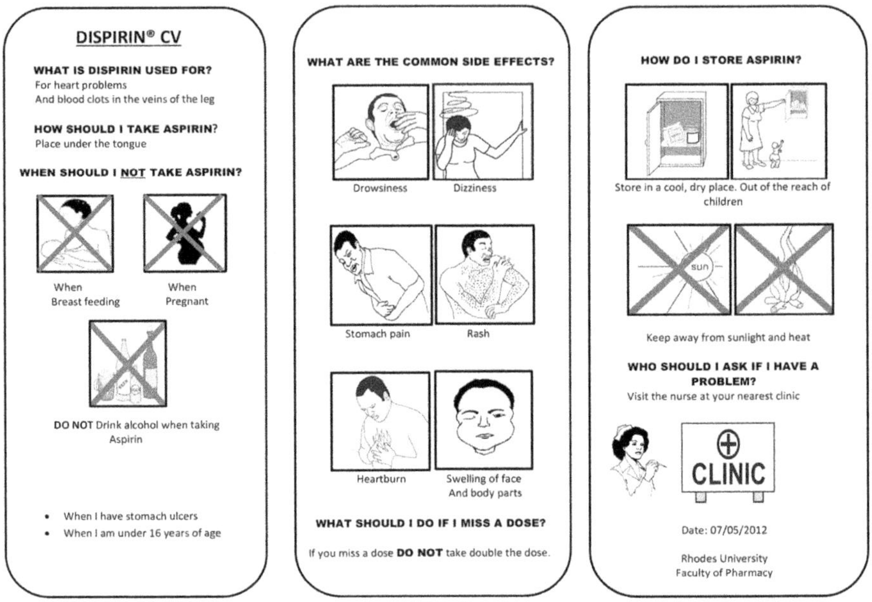

Figure 8.3 Disprin (aspirin) pictographic MIL developed by third-year pharmacy students. Figure by the authors.

Discussion

While the service-learning course was ostensibly undertaken in the form of group work, each student was expected to submit individual self-reflection statements in which they critically accessed their personal development, using one of the CCFOs as a point of discussion. In compiling their research proposals, students were expected to develop the skills required for research-proposal writing, to come to understand the sociocultural context in which the need arose for the development of pictograms to supplement traditional MILs, and to understand the need for the pharmacy profession to respond to the challenge of low health literacy in the South African context. The process of putting their proposals through a formal ethics review impressed upon students the realities and ethical responsibilities of working with real—as opposed to theoretical—population groups. This is an important part of pharmacy education if students are to learn how to perform effective education interventions and to promote healthcare awareness with community members.

Through the consultative drafting process used to design the MILs, students were able to gain deeper insight into the way pictographic MILs operate within the domain of cultural and contextual symbols and representations. Student modifications to the pictographic MILs were made in light of their newfound understanding of how health literacy operates within the domain of the cultural, aesthetic, and symbolic, rather than merely the rational, logical, and linguistic. From a mobilities perspective, pictographic MILs designed with cultural and contextual relevance speak to the important role a sense of place ought to play in the symbols and meanings used for health literacy. MILs themselves must be understood as objects in motion, crossing physical, linguistic, and cultural borders. Following this, it is important to think of them as capturing symbols and meanings that are in flux—adapting to the terrain and surroundings they find themselves in, in order to remain fit for purpose. In working with real patients and the MILs generated with them, students came to see for themselves that "from a *theoretical* point of view human actors encode things with significance, [while] from a *methodological* point of view it is the things-in-motion that illuminate their human and social context" (Appadurai 1986: 5).

Through their consultations with their community participants, students also gained a deeper insight into the practical uses of pictographic MILs and how pictographic MILs would need to be used by pharmacists in dispensing programs that serve populations with low literacy and, in particular, low health literacy. Further, through the development and testing of culturally sensitive and appropriate MILs, students attained an understanding of and appreciation for the positive impacts on the ability of local populations to use medicines rationally that can be made possible through the incorporation of socially and culturally appropriate materials. Here students began to understand how the use of pictographic MILs could improve epistemological and ontological access to healthcare for patients, improving their health literacy and breaking down some of the barriers to effective healthcare that they face. While the sample groups were not comprised of individuals who would receive the final products through their intended channel of distribution (namely, the pictographic MILs distributed by the Phelophepa Trains), these individuals received useful information on commonly used medications.

The inclusion of the critical reflection element in the final report ensured that the practical component of the course was recorded, analyzed, and contextualized within a theoretical framework. This reflective process within a research report allowed students to fully understand the interplay of theory and praxis that was required in the process of designing, testing, and using the pictographic MILs. It also allowed students to reflect on the broader issues underpinning the course in relation to health literacy within a South African context and their role as future pharmacists within this context. Students reported that they gained a deeper understanding of their community healthcare needs and learned valuable skills for ethical interaction with population groups who are typically marginalized or prejudiced against by healthcare workers. Through this service-learning course, students engaged in a process of mobile learning, allowing themselves to be moved as they moved with objects and populations, "participating in their continual shift through time, place and relations with others" (Watts and Urry 2008: 867). The students' experiences here of populations in epistemic and cultural motion, as well as objects and symbols in motion, highlights concretely the ways in which "people are moved by movement" (Salazar et al. 2017: 2).

Primary and universal healthcare promotion is an essential goal of both the Declaration of Alma-Ata (1978) and the WHO Social Determinants of Health (Declaration of Alma-Ata n.d.). In contrast to other developing nations, South Africa faces a unique combination of obstacles in pursuit of this goal. The country's quadruple burden of diseases is exacerbated by low access to healthcare professionals and facilities. As such, service-learning projects tailored to redress specific gaps in the healthcare system while catering to the needs of a community are well positioned to meet several requirements simultaneously, particularly when operating in partnership with national programs such as Phelophepa. Such projects are beneficial to individuals in target communities, where they promote access to healthcare systems, improve health literacy, and enhance patient-healthcare worker relationships. Additionally, students benefit from a holistic educational experience that actively responds to the academic milestones recommended by the CCFOs.

It is imperative for the pharmacy profession, pharmacy educators, and the public health community to investigate, identify, and determine ways in which pharmacists are currently contributing to the shifting space of public health and to determine the extent to which this is reported in the literature. The extent to which pharmacists fulfill public health services has, until recently, not been thoroughly evaluated, and little attention has been paid to this from a mobilities perspective. But pharmacists and pharmacy practices are suitably positioned to provide and promote public health services (Strand et al. 2016), particularly as they move across epistemic and cultural borders that have served to divide and exclude populations from access to healthcare. Developing and sharing accessible health information is only one part of improving health literacy. If interventions are to improve public health, then it is crucial that community-based educational outreach projects adopt strategies that are culturally sensitive and personable in order to empower community members with the confidence to act on their knowledge and to support others to do the same (Nutbeam 2008). If this can be achieved, the possibilities for a variety of mobilities to be enhanced within the healthcare sector could be transformative at a national scale.

Concluding Remarks

In developing countries such as South Africa, the real and pressing need to develop innovative ways to improve the currently ineffective healthcare system—which marginalizes those who move in rural, hard-to-reach populations, in particular—must be met through innovative advancements in access to healthcare and through an increase in the efficacy of available health resources. Innovation within this context does not necessarily imply the introduction of technological advances that rely on population access to, or understanding of, technological equipment such as computers and smartphones. The mobile health clinic Trains described in this chapter remind us that innovation can come through harnessing old technological resources in new ways and putting them to use to meet the needs of underserved populations. These populations can benefit the most from the creative reimagining of existing infrastructure or modes of communication. Initiatives such as the Phelophepa Trains, described in this chapter, are important and uniquely innovative ways to meet the primary healthcare needs of underserved populations whose geographical location—and, more particularly, socioeconomic status—makes accessing healthcare facilities inherently challenging. Though the rail technology may not be new, its use has been reimagined for the public good.

Similarly, in this chapter the authors have described one of the research programs offered by the Phelophepa Trains aimed at improving services, in the form of the development of pictographic MILs for improving the health literacy of patients accessing essential medicines from the Trains—as well as improving communication between pharmacists and low-literate patients who are typically served by the Phelophepa pharmacy. It might at first seem counterintuitive to describe the pictographic MILs discussed in this chapter as technological advances aimed at improving health, given that they are not as obviously high-tech as those advances typically discussed in current literature. However, these pictographic MILs constitute technologies that improve the health literacy of the patients for whom they are designed and force us to rethink what advances are required in designing technologies for global health initiatives that are most effective—particularly for advancing the healthcare needs of the poor and underserved populations.

Campus-based work at universities that collaborate with Phelophepa, such as those described in this chapter, are essential not only for improving the level of training for university students provided onboard the Trains during their service, but for improving the level of primary healthcare provided by Phelophepa. More generally, such collaborative work is essential for improving the overall performance of the South African healthcare system, which can benefit from research that focuses on addressing context-specific, culturally sensitive community-related healthcare challenges, as well as for equipping the next generation of healthcare workers to be more aware of and responsive to a broader range of societal healthcare needs.

Acknowledgments

The authors acknowledge the third-year pharmacy students who completed this group research in producing the MILs pictured in this chapter. Ms Wendy Wrench is acknowledged for her critical role in representing the Faculty of Pharmacy on the Phelophepa Train and assessing the final drafts of the MILs. Associate professor emeritus Ros Dowse is acknowledged for the once-off session held each year to appraise students on important techniques in designing MILs. Dr Carmen Oltmann is acknowledged for the once-off session each year highlighting aspects related to ethics in research.

Sunitha C. Srinivas, PhD, began an academic career at Rhodes University founded strongly on her experiences as the provincial technical coordinator of the Delhi Society for the Promotion of Rational Use of Drugs and the India-World Health Organization Essential Medicines Program. She is a recipient of the Vice Chancellor's Community Engagement Award (2008) and the Internationalization Award (2014) from Rhodes University and a recipient of the Association of Commonwealth Universities Titular Fellowship (2011), South Africa's National Excellence in Teaching and Learning Award (2014), and the Tallories Network's University Education for Transformative Leadership in Africa Mini Grant in 2015 for Community Engagement.

Sharli Anne Paphitis, PhD, is a South African philosopher and community engagement practitioner who received her doctorate in philosophy from Rhodes University. She has lectured in applied ethics, philosophy, community engaged learning, and service learning at Rhodes University and the University of Fort Hare. She was an Andrew Mellon, NRF, and Erasmus doctoral scholar and the recipient of the Rhodes University Vice Chancellor's Distinguished Award for Community Engagement. Her research has focused largely on personal autonomy, identity, human agency, and epistemic justice. She has tried to bring this philosophical work to bear on her approach to community engagement, focusing on human development in engaged learning projects she has established and cofacilitated at Rhodes University.

REFERENCES

American Friends of the Phelophepa Train. 2015. "Train of Hope." New York: American Friends of the Phelophepa Train. Retrieved 31 August 2016 from https://www.trainofhope.org/.

Appadurai, A. 1986. *The Social Life of Things: Commodities in Cultural Perspective.* Cambridge: Cambridge University Press.

Baker, D. W. 2006. "The Meaning and the Measure of Health Literacy." *Journal of General Internal Medicine* 21(8): 878–83.

Bann, C. M., L. A. McCormack, N. D. Berkman, and L. B. Squiers. 2012. "The Health Literacy Skills Instrument: A 10-Item Short Form." *Journal of Health Communication* 17(Suppl. 3): 191–202.

Bassett, I. V., D. Govindasamy, A. S. Erlwanger, E. P. Hyle, K. Kranzer, N. van Schaik, F. Noubary, et al. 2014. "Mobile HIV Screening in Cape Town, South Africa: Clinical Impact, Cost and Cost-Effectiveness." *PLoS ONE* 9(1). doi:10.1371/journal.pone.0085197.

Benatar, S. 2013. "The Challenges of Health Disparities in South Africa." *South African Medical Journal* 103(3): 154–55.

Benjamin, E., L. Swartz, L. Hering, and B. Chilza. 2016. "Language Barriers in Health: Lessons from the Experiences of Trained Interpreters Working in Public Sector Hospitals in the Western Cape." In *South African Health Review 2016,* ed. A. Padarath, J. King, E. Mackie, and J. Casciola, 17–24. Durban: Health Systems Trust. Retrieved 31 August 2016 from https://www.health-e.org.za/wp-content/uploads/2016/05/South-African-Health-Review-2016.pdf.

Bhayat, A., G. Vergotine, V. Yengopal, and M. J. Rudolph. 2011. "The Impact of Service-Learning on Two Groups of South African Dental Students." *Journal of Dental Education* 75(11): 1482–8.

Center on an Aging Society. 2004. "Cultural Competence in Health Care." Issue Brief No. 5, February. Center on an Aging Society, Georgetown University. Retrieved 31 August 2016 from https://georgetown.app.box.com/s/0ttelx2xtn3wyzc7kmlb.

Declaration of Alma-Ata. 1978. International Conference on Primary Health Care, Alma-Ata, USSR, 6–12 September. Retrieved 31 August 2016 from http://www.who.int/publications/almaata_declaration_en.pdf.

Dowse, R., and M. Ehlers. 2001. "The Evaluation of Pharmaceutical Pictograms in a Low-Literate South African Population." *Patient Education and Counseling* 45(2): 87–99.

Dowse, R., and M. Ehlers. 2005. "Medicine Labels Incorporating Pictograms: Do They Influence Understanding and Adherence?" *Patient Education and Counseling* 58(1): 63–70.

Hagan, S., L. Swartz, S. Kilian, B. Chiliza, P. Bisogno, and J. Joska. 2013. "The Accuracy of Interpreting Key Psychiatric Terms by Ad Hoc Interpreters at a South African Psychiatric Hospital." *African Journal of Psychiatry* 16(6): 424–29.

Hansraj, R. 2009. "The Perspective of Optometry Students of the Phelophepa Train regarding Its Role in Developing Experiential Skills." *South African Optometrist* 68(2): 61–69.

Hill, C., D. Zurakowski, J. Bennet, R. Walker-White, J. L. Osman, A. Quarles, and N. Oriol. 2012. "Knowledgeable Neighbors: A Mobile Clinic Model for Disease Prevention and Screening in Underserved Communities." *American Journal of Public Health* 102(3): 406–10.

Jacobs, A. C., M. J. MacKenzie, and Y. Botma. 2013. "Learning Experiences of Student Nurses on a Healthcare Train in the Free State Province of South Africa." *Africa Journal of Nursing and Midwifery* 15(1): 3–14.

Jacobs, L. 2004. "The Tracks of Healing." *Journal of the Royal Society for the Promotion of Health* 124(4): 159.

Kagee, A., R. H. Remiem, A. Berkman, S. Hoffman, L. Campos, and L. Swartz. 2011. "Structural Barriers to ART Adherence in Southern Africa: Challenges and Potential Ways Forward." *Global Public Health* 6(1): 83–97.

Koodibetse, K. G. 2015. "HIV/AIDS Stigma and Discrimination in South Africa – Still a Problem." *South African Medical Journal* 105(9): 703.

Maheswaran, H., H. Thulare, D. Stanistreet, F. Tanser, and M. L. Newell. 2012. "Starting a Home and Mobile HIV Testing Service in a Rural Area of South Africa." *Journal of Acquired Immune Deficiency Syndromes* 59(3): e43–e46. doi:10.1097/QAI.0b013e3182414ed7.

McLaren, Z., C. Ardington, and M. Leibbrandt. 2013. "Distance as a Barrier to Health Care Access in South Africa." Working Paper. Southern Africa Labour and Development Research Unit, University of Cape Town. Retrieved 31 August 2016 from http://www.opensaldru.uct.ac.za/handle/11090/613.

Miller, M. J., H. B. Degenholtz, J. A. Gazmararian, C. J. Lin, E. M. Ricci, and S. M. Sereika. 2007. "Identifying Elderly at Greatest Risk of Inadequate Health Literacy: A Predictive Model for Population-Health Decision Makers." *Research in Social and Administrative Pharmacy* 3(1): 70–85.

Naidoo, P., K. Peltzer, J. Louw, G. Matseke, G. Mchunu, and B. Tutshana. 2013. "Predictors of Tuberculosis (TB) and Antiretroviral (ARV) Medication Non-Adherence in Public Primary Care Patients in South Africa: A Cross Sectional Study." *BMC Public Health* 13: 396.

South Africa. National Department of Health. 1996. *National Drug Policy for South Africa.* Pretoria: National Department of Health. Retrieved 31 August 2016 from http://apps.who.int/medicinedocs/documents/s17744en/s17744en.pdf.

South Africa. National Department of Health. 2011. Policy on Language Services for the National Department of Health. Pretoria: National Department of Health. Retrieved 31 August 2016 from http://pmg-assets.s3-website-eu-west-1.amazonaws.com/150527healthlanguagepolicy.pdf.

Nutbeam, D. 2008. "The Evolving Concept of Health Literacy." *Social Science & Medicine* 67(12): 2072–8.

Oriol, N. E., P. J. Cote, A. P. Vavasis, J. Bennet, D. DeLorenzo, P. Blanc, and I. Kohane. 2009. "Calculating the Return on Investment of Mobile Healthcare." *BMC Medicine* 7: 27. doi:10.1186/1741-7015-7-27.

Pleasant, A. 2013. "Health Literacy around the World: Part 1. Health Literacy Efforts Outside of the United States." In IOM (Institute of Medicine), *Health Literacy: Im-*

proving Health, Health Systems, and Health Policy around the World: Workshop Summary, Appendix A. Washington, DC: National Academies Press. Retrieved 31 August 2016 from http://www.ncbi.nlm.nih.gov/books/NBK202445/.

Raynor, D. K. 2013. "User Testing in Developing Patient Medication Information in Europe." *Research in Social and Administrative Pharmacy* 9(5): 640–45.

Rispel, L. 2016. "Analysing the Progress and Fault Lines of Health Sector Transformation in South Africa." In *South African Health Review 2016,* ed. A. Padarath, J. King, E. Mackie, and J. Casciola, 17–24. Durban: Health Systems Trust. Retrieved 31 August 2016 from https://www.health-e.org.za/wp-content/uploads/2016/05/South-African-Health-Review-2016.pdf.

Salazar, N. B., A. Elliot, and R. Norum. 2017. "Studying Mobilities: Theoretical Notes and Methodological Queries." In *Methodologies of Mobility: Ethnography and Experiment,* ed. A. Elliot, R. Norum, and N. B. Salazar, 1–24. Oxford: Berghahn Books.

SAQA (South African Qualifications Authority). 2000. *The National Qualifications Framework and Curriculum Development.* Pretoria: Department of Education. Retrieved 31 August 2016 from http://www.saqa.org.za/docs/pol/2000/curriculum_dev.pdf.

Sheller, M., and J. Urry. 2006. "The New Mobilities Paradigm." *Environment and Planning A* 38(2): 207–26.

Sheridan, S. L., D. J. Halpern, A. J. Viera, N. D. Berkman, K. E. Donahue, and K. Crotty. 2011. "Interventions for Individuals with Low Health Literacy: A Systematic Review." *Journal of Health Communication* 16(Suppl. 3): 30–54.

Sørensen, K., J. M. Pelikan, F. Röthlin, K. Ganahl, Z. Slonska, G. Doyle, J. Fullam, et al. 2015. "Health Literacy in Europe: Comparative Results of the European Health Literacy Survey (HLS-EU)." *European Journal of Public Health* 25(6): 1053–8.

Strand, M. A., J. Tellers, A. Patterson, A. Ross, and L. Palombi. 2016. "The Achievement of Public Health Services in Pharmacy Practice: A Literature Review." *Research in Social and Administrative Pharmacy* 12(2): 247–56.

Tanser, F., B. Gijsbertsen, and K. Herbst. 2006. "Modeling and Understanding Primary Health Care Accessibility and Utilization in Rural South Africa: An Exploration Using a Geographical Information System." *Social Science & Medicine* 63(3): 691–705.

Truter, I. 2010. "The Phelophepa Health Care Train: A Pharmacoepidemiological Overview of the Western Cape in 2009." *South African Family Practice* 52(5): 463–66.

———. 2013. "Experiential Learning Experience of Pharmacy Students on the Phelophepa Health Care Train." *Jordan Journal of Pharmaceutical Sciences* 6(2): 171–78.

Van Dyk, A. C. 2011. "Antiretroviral Adherence in South Africa: Are We Burning Our Bridges?" Inaugural Lecture. University of South Africa. Retrieved 31 August 2016 from http://uir.unisa.ac.za/bitstream/handle/10500/4970/Van%20Dyk%20Inaugural%20Lecture%2026%20Okt%202011.pdf.

Vos, J., M. W. Borgdorff, and E. G. Kachidza. 1990. "Cost and Output of Mobile Clinics in a Commercial Farming Area in Zimbabwe." *Social Science & Medicine* 31(11): 1207–11.

Wali, H., and K. Grindrod. 2016. "Don't Assume the Patient Understands: Qualitative Analysis of the Challenges Low Health Literate Patients Face in the Pharmacy." *Research in Social and Administrative Pharmacy.* Retrieved 31 August 2016 from https://

www.researchgate.net/publication/289497196_Don't_assume_the_patient_unde rstands_Qualitative_analysis_of_the_challenges_low_health_literate_patients_face _in_the_pharmacy.

Watts, L., and J. Urry. 2008. "Moving Methods, Travelling Times." *Environment and Planning D: Society and Space* 26(5): 860–74.

WHO (World Health Organization). 2014. *Global Tuberculosis Control 2014.* Geneva: WHO. Retrieved 31 August 2016 from http://apps.who.int/iris/bitstream/10665/137094/1/9789241564809_eng.pdf.

Wong, S. 2012. "Health Literacy Programs for Older Adults: A Systematic Literature Review." *Health Education Research* 27(6): 947–60.

CHAPTER 9

Community-Led Peer Advocacy for Transgender Healthcare Access in the Southeastern United States

The Trans Buddy Program

E. Kale Edmiston

Transgender Southerners and Movement in Public Space

The US South is generally considered a culturally conservative region (Woodberry and Smith 1998). As such, transgender people in the US South may find themselves in a hostile climate (Hasenbush et al. 2014), one in which increased visibility does not necessarily lead to improved quality of life. In many ways, increased visibility may in fact increase harm for transgender people, particularly transgender women, trans feminine people, and gender-nonconforming people. A recent study indicates that when transgender people are perceived by others to be visibly transgender, they are more likely to experience violence and discrimination, and are also more likely to engage in coping mechanisms that have a negative impact on health, such as alcohol abuse and tobacco use (Miller and Grollman 2015). Estimates indicate a more than fourfold increase in the murder rate for transgender women compared with that of the overall female population (Stotzer 2009; Human Rights Campaign 2016). Furthermore, more transgender people were murdered in 2015 than in any year since statistics have been gathered, the overwhelming majority of them young transgender women of color; one-third of these reported murders were of women living in the South. Because Southern regional politics so often involve fear-mongering regarding lesbian, gay, bisexual, and transgender (LGBT) individuals, increased contact with LGBT people does not actually lead to improved attitudes in the South as it may in other regions (Barth and Overby 2003). Additionally, transgender people and allies must now combat antitransgender legislation that attempts to restrict their movement in public spaces. This type of legislation has swept many states in the southeastern United States; one example is North Carolina's HB2 legislation that would require transgender people to use restrooms and other public facilities that align with their genitalia rather than with their lived gender (Herman, Mallory, and Wilson 2016). Many of the issues facing transgender people nationally, but particularly in the South, are at their foundation about mobility in public spaces and the health consequences of restricted mobility.

Many transgender people have limited access to public spaces, including restrooms, airports, voter polling locations, healthcare facilities, locker rooms, and public schools and universities (Cotton 2012; Currah and Mulqueen 2011). When transgender people are able to access public spaces, they often face extraordinarily high rates of violence, including harassment on public transportation and in clinical waiting rooms (Grant et al. 2011). Limited access to public space, as well as travel barriers to these spaces, is a product of social and economic marginalization caused by transphobia. Limited access and mobility in public spaces has long-term consequences for the health of transgender people (Poteat, German, and Kerrigan 2013). Employment and housing discrimination, difficulty accessing identification documents, and policies and practices that either assume cisgender identity (a cisgender person is one whose gender identity aligns with the sex they were assigned at birth) or overtly exclude transgender people create situations wherein transgender people, particularly those who are disabled or people of color, are more likely to experience violence and poverty and less likely to access healthcare (Lombardi et al. 2001; Mananzala and Spade 2007; White-Hughto, Reisner, and Pachankis 2015).

Healthcare access is linked to barriers to mobility and safe public spaces available for transgender people. Previous work in populations that travel to access healthcare, such as migrant populations, has shown that individuals may opt to travel to access care due to unequal distribution of healthcare resources or to access care that is culturally competent (Ellis and Muschkin 1996). For example, a study of migration of HIV-positive individuals living in the rural South and traveling to urban clinics found that most participants had acquired their infection locally and did not relocate following transmission. Rural-dwelling residents were also less likely than urban-dwelling individuals to relocate following diagnosis. Here, the authors highlight the importance of HIV prevention and treatment interventions designed to meet the needs of individuals living in the rural South, who have less mobility and fewer resources than people who live in urban areas (Agee et al. 2007). Limited mobility—due to travel costs, lack of a means of travel (or safe means of travel), or lack of information about available healthcare resources—results in barriers to healthcare (Vindrola-Padros and Johnson 2015). *Hence, many transgender people find themselves needing to travel to access healthcare providers with experience treating transgender patients, but less likely to be able to do so.* People who must travel to access healthcare are less likely to be care adherent, more likely to seek treatment late, and less likely to have social support to assist in health maintenance (Tanser et al. 2015). When limited mobility is coupled with social marginalization's negative lifetime impact on health, the net effect is extreme isolation and poor health outcomes (Mao et al. 2015). Despite this, there has been virtually no discussion in the mobility literature of the access barriers faced by transgender people in the US South. Given this gap in the literature, this chapter situates transgender healthcare access in the context of the mobility literature: a novel approach to considering transgender health inequality.

Transgender Health Disparities

Transgender people as a population experience poorer health outcomes than cisgender people (Institute of Medicine 2011). Importantly, a growing body of literature on health disparity in transgender populations addresses how limited access to care creates and perpetuates health disparities (for a review, see Safer et al. 2016). However, the majority of this literature focuses on the experiences of urban-dwelling transgender people living in coastal cities, particularly New York, San Francisco, Boston, and Los Angeles (for a review, see Edmiston et al. 2016). The National Transgender Discrimination Survey reports that 28 percent of transgender people delay care due to fears of discrimination and that 30 percent of transgender people experience violence or harassment at their provider's office. State-specific data about the experiences of transgender people suggest higher rates of violence and health disparity in the US South than in other regions of the United States (Grant et al. 2011). Although the interpersonal bias and discrimination that transgender people may encounter in healthcare settings certainly contributes to delay of care and poor health outcomes, systemic marginalization and transphobia also plays a critical role in perpetuating health disparity (Roberts and Fantz 2014). For example, people who are unable to access proper identification—and are therefore less able to access transportation, education, employment, and housing—will have poorer health outcomes. Unsurprisingly, transgender people living in poverty and without health insurance are more likely to delay care (Cruz 2014). For people living in regions with fewer resources, these disparities are compounded.

The overall population of the US South has higher rates of poverty (CDC 2013a), lower rates of health insurance coverage (DeNavas-Walt, Proctor, and Smith 2011), higher rates of chronic illnesses (CDC 2013a), and a lower average life expectancy (CDC 2013b) than other regions in the United States. The reasons for these regional health disparities are complex, but healthcare policy, cultural values, city planning, and the built environment have all been suggested as possible causes (CDC 2013a). The few studies to address health disparity among LGBT people living in the South suggest that health disparities are magnified for LGBT Southerners. An estimated one in four LGBT people living in the US South do not have health insurance, and 28 percent of LGBT Southerners report not having enough money to pay for healthcare (Hasenbush et al. 2014). The South is home to many of the most marginalized LGBT people. LGBT Southerners are more likely to be Black, have lower educational attainment (in contrast to LGBT people living in other regions, who tend to have higher educational attainment than heterosexual people), and are more likely to live in poverty than LGBT people in other regions of the United States (Hasenbush et al. 2014). There have been almost no public or behavioral health studies specifically of transgender people in rural areas or transgender people in the US South (for a review, see Edmiston et al. 2016). To date, only one study has focused on the experiences of transgender Southerners—the results of which indicate profound challenges. In this Virginia-based survey study, 38 percent of respondents were living at or below the poverty line. Over 40 percent of respondents reported experiencing discrimination, fewer than half were out as transgender to their primary care provider, and more than 25 percent were not able to access transgender-related healthcare services in the last month. In terms of behavioral health measures, 64 percent reported lifetime tobacco use and 23 percent reported having a problem with alcohol use. Twenty-seven percent report a lifetime history of rape, 38 percent reported having experienced a physical attack, and 31 percent did not have supportive families. Transgender people who were a racial or ethnic minority and who had low income or low educational attainment were more likely to report discrimination (Bradford et al. 2013).

Only one study to date has compared transgender people living in rural areas with those in urban areas, finding more severe mental illness symptoms among transgender men living in rural areas than among those living in urban areas, as well as high rates of unprotected sex among transgender women and binge drinking among both transgender men and transgender women regardless of urban or rural location (Horvath et al. 2014). There is an obvious need for more research that addresses health disparities specific to transgender people living in rural areas and in the US South. The small extant literature suggests that health disparities are extreme and are related to significant experiences with violence, stigma, and marginalization. Such experiences limit the mobility of transgender people in public space and their ability to move freely through the world without fear.

Outside of the public health literature, there has been very little qualitative research on the experiences of transgender people seeking healthcare. These studies have found that healthcare remains a significant challenge for transgender people, seen particularly in a lack of provider and support staff knowledge or education about transgender issues (James-Abra et al. 2015; McCann 2015; McCann and Sharek 2014). The experiences of transgender people in the South, particularly in rural areas, remain largely within-community knowledge, but it is likely that the struggles transgender people face are more pronounced for Southerners and compounded by additional challenges that are unique to the South.

Within-Community Solutions to Mobility and Access Challenges

Because most Southern cities and rural communities do not have the population density to support LGBT-specific medical clinics or services, transgender Southerners have created information and support networks to access healthcare (Schrock, Holden, and Reid 2004). These survival strategies exist in other regional transgender communities (Roller, Sedlak, and Draucker 2015), but may be of particular necessity for rural and Southern transgender people. These strategies include the creation of informal lists that are shared within the community for transgender-affirming (or even transgender-tolerant) health and personal care services, including transition-related healthcare, gynecologists, psychiatrists, hair and nail salons, and gyms. The presence of such lists in nearly every Southern community underscores the extent to which the mobility of transgender people is limited in public spaces—some transgender people do not even feel safe scheduling a haircut without first accessing a referral network to ensure they will not experience violence. Furthermore, low population density limits the size of transgender communities in a given area (particularly in less populous rural areas). When coupled with the small pool of providers with experience seeing transgender people who are also willing to see transgender patients or provide transition-related care (Khalili, Leung, and Diamant 2015), many transgender Southerners must travel for hours, even out of state, to access basic medical care in an affirming environment. In this context, it is unsurprising that many transgender people find themselves without options for accessing healthcare, or that many opt to postpone or delay care when accessing healthcare is expensive, is time consuming, and involves significant travel and stress.

What happens when transgender people are able to access care? As stated previously, the majority of transgender Southerners do not have access to LGBT-specific clinics, which are more commonplace in large cities in other regions such as San Francisco, Los Angeles, Chicago, Philadelphia, New York, and Boston. As a result, transgender people in the South must learn to travel through healthcare systems that were not designed for them. This lack of consideration is apparent to transgender people from the waiting room to the exam table. For example, although more clinics have begun to address the limitations of standard intake forms, most forms do not allow transgender people to describe their identities, bodies, or health needs (Conron, Scout, and Austin 2008). There is also significant lack of provider knowledge about the purpose of gender-inclusive intake forms (Carabez et al. 2015). Restroom facilities are likely sex-segregated. Most electronic medical record (EMR) systems do not allow providers to accurately record their patients' identities, leading to gaps in continuity of care (Cahill et al. 2014). Sex-specific billing codes and insurance policy line-item exclusions create challenges for patients and providers when interfacing with insurance companies and Medicare (Green 2014). These obstacles exist even in situations where providers and support staff are well informed, professional, and supportive of transgender patients, highlighting the systemic nature of transphobic bias in healthcare institutions (Snelgrove et al. 2012). Such systemic transphobia is often a "roadblock" that limits transgender patients' ability to travel through healthcare settings, be it the waiting room, the restroom, or the exam room.

The Trans Buddy Approach to Healthcare Support

The Trans Buddy Program was founded in Nashville, Tennessee, in 2014 to provide support for transgender people seeking healthcare in recognition of the systemic and interpersonal barriers they face when accessing healthcare. The Trans Buddy Program provides transgender patients seeking care with trained peer advocates who are available by phone or to attend healthcare visits with transgender clients. Peer advocates offer transgender individuals phone and in-person support, including healthcare referrals and resources. Transgender peer advocates, or "Trans Buddies," also attend transgender community events and, by request, healthcare appointments. In this regard, the Trans Buddy Program represents an innovative and intentionally low-tech solution to the access and mobility challenges faced by transgender people in the US South. The goal of the program is to improve healthcare access and care adherence for transgender people by facilitating communication between clinical care teams and transgender patients, and by providing patients with resources to make informed and empowered healthcare decisions.

Many Trans Buddy clients live in the rural areas, are elderly, or are disabled. Other clients may work at nearby military bases. These clients have limited access to transgender culture and community for many reasons: their mobility may be limited by distance from and lack of transportation to major cities where transgender culture is more visible and accessible. They may not have the financial resources to travel to urban centers on a regular basis or have high-speed Internet to access online transgender communities. They may have increased need for privacy when accessing transgender support services due to fears of losing their job, and therefore cannot attend public events or support group meetings. Because of these challenges, the Trans Buddy Program's approach is deliberately low-tech. By using a phone hotline model, the program can ensure greater accessibility of the service to transgender people whose mobility or financial resources are limited. Furthermore, because many people living in rural areas do not have access to high-speed Internet, the use of a phone hotline model is more accessible to a larger number of people. As a result, many of the clients who utilize our services call to ask a specific question about a healthcare referral, but remain on the line in order to talk to a supportive person (be they cisgender or transgender). Although our Trans Buddy volunteers are not qualified to give medical advice, they are trained to listen with compassion. Many clients end up asking questions about transition that they may be afraid to ask in person, as well as questions about dating, sexuality, and the coming-out process.

Trans Buddy volunteers also attend healthcare appointments with transgender clients. Such appointments are always at the client's discretion and can result from a specific request by a client via the phone hotline for an upcoming scheduled appointment or for emergent or inpatient care. Providers can also request a Trans Buddy on behalf of a patient, with the patient's permission. For scheduled care visits, Trans Buddies are encouraged to discuss the details of the visit with clients beforehand to facilitate communication about goals, concerns, and desired outcomes for the healthcare encounter. Regardless of the situation, Trans Buddies are there to support their clients, facilitate communication between clients, providers, and staff, and assist clients as they move through the medical system, from intake to aftercare.

The Trans Buddy Approach to Client Mobility

There are a number of ways that Trans Buddy volunteers can improve client mobility and access in the healthcare setting (see Figure 9.1). In thinking about movement through healthcare clinics and hospitals, the concept of micromobility is useful. Micromobility takes the concepts of mobility research and applies them to the individual (Gutierrez 2008). This concept allows us to examine how systems that were not designed for transgender people impact their mobility and, therefore, their access to healthcare resources (Vindrola-Padros and Johnson 2015). Hospitals, as institutions and literal spaces, exist at the intersection of public and private. The evolution of healthcare technologies and the changing orientation of hospitals from charitable institutions to centers for education and sites of biomedical research has certainly impacted the experiences of both providers and patients, as well as the character of provider-patient interactions (Finkler, Hunter, and Iedema 2008).

For transgender people, this changing healthcare landscape has several unique consequences, which Trans Buddy advocates can begin to address.

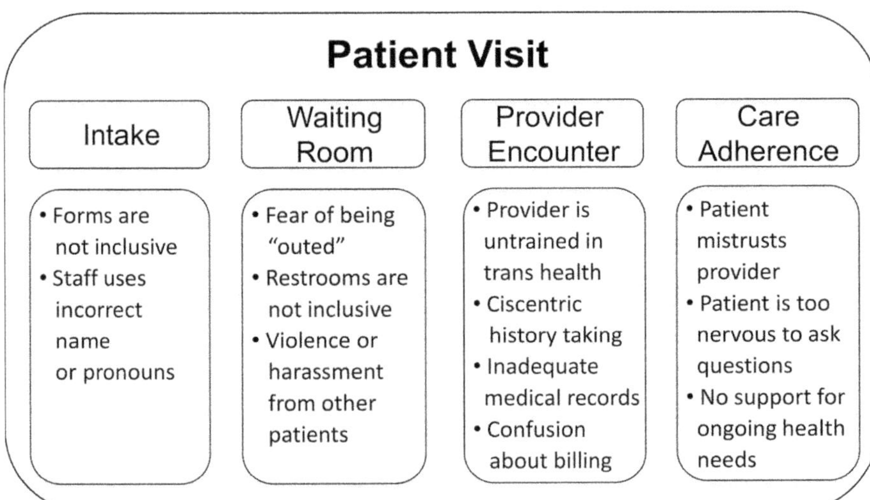

Figure 9.1 Transphobic healthcare systems limit mobility and access. Figure by the author.

For example, at intake, Trans Buddy volunteers can help clients by answering questions about forms that may assume cisgender identity. In the waiting room, volunteers can help clients generate lists of questions they may want to ask the provider or offer emotional support to a client experiencing anxiety or distress. In the instance of sex-segregated facilities, such as women's clinics, or procedures related to natal pelvic anatomy, Trans Buddy volunteers can serve as a "beard" for transgender people who may appear to be in the "wrong" place (e.g., a transgender male client may request a female Trans Buddy volunteer for a pelvic exam appointment so that other patients will assume the Trans Buddy volunteer is the patient, thereby avoiding stares or potential harassment in the waiting room). Trans Buddies can also communicate with intake staff to ensure that the appropriate name is used when the client is called for their appointment. This allows the client to avoid the stress and possible violent repercussions of being misgendered or outed publicly. Finally, as most restroom facilities are sex-segregated, Trans Buddy volunteers may enter the restroom with a client at their request to ensure they will not be harassed. Thus, much of the work of Trans Buddy volunteers is centered on improving clients' movement through healthcare facilities.

As the client moves from the waiting room to the exam room, Trans Buddy volunteers are trained to advocate for their client while also facilitating communication with their provider. Given that trust and clear communication between provider and patient are primary determinants of care adherence (Rosen 2014), Trans Buddy volunteers have the potential to improve health outcomes. In practice, the role of the Trans Buddy can range from quietly holding a client's hand while they undergo an anxiety-provoking procedure, taking notes regarding aftercare or medication side effects, or reminding their client to ask about generic medications to reduce costs. Trans Buddy volunteers also frequently answer provider questions about ICD-10 billing codes, local transgender resources, and professional society guidelines for the care of transgender patients. In such situations, Trans Buddy volunteers are trained to engage their client in all conversations. For example, if a provider asks a question about charting gender identity, the Trans Buddy volunteer will explain various options and the relative benefits of each approach, then ask the client and the provider to develop a solution together for how to identify the patient in their EMR. The presence of Trans Buddy volunteers has facilitated access for the program's clients and improved healthcare utilization and provider communication. Many of our transgender clients as well as providers who frequently see transgender patients have requested our service multiple times. Although no research has specifically investigated outcomes related to peer advocacy in transgender populations, research on the positive impact of health coaches and other advocates who do not have specific medical training has indicated positive outcomes in terms of healthcare access and utilization (Ellis et al. 2015). Thus, Trans Buddy volunteers have the potential to make a significant positive impact on the health of transgender people.

In addition to assisting with healthcare appointments, the Trans Buddy Program also plays a key role in improving local transgender mobility and access to resources. Because transgender communities in the South may be small or distributed over wide geographic areas, the Trans Buddy Program facilitates connection among transgender people by acting as a "resource hub." This service was inspired by the long-standing and continuing practice of transgender support groups—groups that often generate lists of transgender-friendly providers and services, as discussed previously. However, because the transgender community is diverse with respect to race, age, socioeconomic status, immigration status, ability, and educational attainment, these lists alone cannot serve the needs of every transgender person (Jann, Edmiston, and Ehrenfeld 2015). Because the Trans Buddy Program operates at the level of the client-volunteer relationship, volunteers are able to make referrals that will best serve the needs of each client. Furthermore, because Trans Buddy volunteers develop relationships with multiple healthcare institutions and providers, they are well suited to identify the optimal referral. For example, a client who is a sex worker, does not have insurance, and needs primary care may be best served by a different provider than a client with access to insurance in a less stigmatized profession who needs primary care. Similarly, a transgender woman who is HIV positive and on Medicaid will have different healthcare needs than a nonbinary person in their twenties who needs a pelvic exam (Roche and Keith 2014). As a result, the Trans Buddy Program's referral and resource list is a living document that reflects the experiences of every client and every volunteer. Transgender people and providers frequently contact us with referrals and recommendations, allowing our list to continually grow. Our approach, which focuses on the client-volunteer relationship, allows us to think systemically and intersectionally while acting to serve the needs of individuals.

Building Relationships to Support Mobility

The Trans Buddy Program's success is largely driven by relationships with existing community organizations. These include transgender support groups, sliding-scale clinics, and HIV/AIDS nonprofits. For example, with their client's permission, Trans Buddy volunteers are able to put rural-dwelling transgender people in touch with support group members who may live near them to provide transportation to meetings. Relationships with key providers have led to expanded, mandatory transgender competency trainings for entire hospital staffs, as well as a slow but steady increase in the number of providers in the region willing to provide transition-related medical care (which decreases the travel burden for individual patients). The Trans Buddy Program has invited healthcare providers to transgender support group meetings so that transgender community members can ask questions and learn about options for transition-related care. Increasingly, the Trans Buddy Program also operates as a training institute in addition to a direct care service. We have connected nurses with transgender youth support groups to provide trainings for parents of transgender children on safe injection techniques for hormones; our volunteers have given structural and cultural competency trainings for clinical students; and Trans Buddy Program leadership has partnered with a small group of providers to create the region's first support group for HIV positive transgender people. Trans Buddy volunteers also attend local meetings of PFLAG (formerly known as Parents, Families, and Friends of Lesbians and Gays), which has largely become a support group for the parents of transgender youth. As parents of transgender youth grapple with their child's identity, Trans Buddy volunteers can serve as ideal models of transgender support and acceptance, while also providing nonjudgmental support for parents who are just learning about transgender identity. As the visibility of our program has grown, so has our reach. Clients from across the South have utilized our service and affiliated support groups, including clients who have driven from several states away to access informed consent cross-gender hormone therapy with a Trans Buddy volunteer by their side. Ideally, travel across such extreme distances should not be necessary to access medically necessary care; we hope that our program can serve as a model for other transgender peer advocacy programs so that all transgender people can access the care they deserve.

Finally, it is important to emphasize that the main determinant of the Trans Buddy Program's success has been the dedicated group of transgender and cisgender leaders, volunteers, and providers who make our program possible. Our program leadership is a diverse group of transgender people and heterosexual or LGB cisgender allies who have worked tirelessly to connect transgender communities with resources and to expand the Trans Buddy Program to multiple hospitals and clinics in the area. Diverse transgender leadership is critical to building trust in our program among local transgender communities. The Trans Buddy Program's transgender leadership—diverse with respect to race, age, gender identity/expression, sexual orientation, disability, and socioeconomic status—makes outreach possible in local transgender communities, particularly communities that experience multiple forms of marginalization. Our cisgender leadership is also critical: they provide an ideal model of cisgender allyship for our partnered organizations and clinics; they may have a larger capacity than our transgender volunteers for helping other cisgender people to challenge their own transphobia; and they may have access to more institutional resources than many transgender people. Our volunteer advocates are also diverse with regards to race and ethnicity, educational attainment, gender identity and expression, sexual orientation, ability, age, and socioeconomic status. This diversity of perspectives has strengthened and enriched our program by allowing us to continually improve our volunteer trainings based on participant feedback, while also allowing a diverse group of transgender clients to feel safe utilizing our program. Specifically, a dedicated group of transgender elders has opted to volunteer with the Trans Buddy Program. This intergenerational transgender community has been a great source of strength and healing for both our clients and our volunteers. Partnership between cisgender and transgender people is the core of what makes the Trans Buddy Program effective.

Taken together, the Trans Buddy Program's services aid the mobility of transgender people by creating access to healthcare and facilitating movement through the healthcare system and healthcare facilities. Volunteers also operate a call line that may help to reduce the need for travel for individuals who are geographically or socially isolated or disabled. The Trans Buddy Program also partners with a variety of existing service organizations, thereby improving access and mobility for transgender people via resource referrals and provider training partnerships.

Access to transition-related care improves the safety and mobility of transgender people in public spaces. Ideally, transgender people would be safe and welcome in all spaces regardless of their transition status or the degree to which they conform to cisgender standards of appearance. However, this is often not the case, and the ability to access hormones, electrolysis, and surgery for those transgender people who want such interventions can mean the difference between safely moving in public spaces and encountering violence. This is increasingly clear as Southern states have enacted or are considering legislation that restricts the mobility of transgender people in public facilities, presumably with the assumption that transgender people are readily recognizable as transgender. Furthermore, transition-related care is associated with improved mental health (Wilson et al. 2015). Improving mental health increases mobility by providing the capacity to engage with public life and public spaces. Finally, because the primary goal of the Trans Buddy Program is to empower transgender patients to make their own healthcare decisions, we ultimately see a ripple effect in which our clients are able to feel more empowered in other aspects of their lives. Our goal is that increased self-efficacy will result in a local transgender community that is less isolated, more connected, and better able to advocate for their needs.

Conclusion

The Trans Buddy Program is a unique peer advocacy program designed to improve healthcare access for transgender people. In the US South and in rural areas, barriers to healthcare can be linked to the unequal distribution of transgender healthcare resources, which creates an increased need for mobility. Furthermore, by applying the concept of micromobility to this population, we can see the ways in which the assumption of cisgender identity limits the mobility of transgender people through the healthcare system, and the ways in which transphobic violence limits safe travel through public space. The Trans Buddy Program seeks to address these problems by pairing transgender people seeking healthcare with peer advocates who can facilitate mobility through public spaces and healthcare systems. One of the key lessons from this program has been the extent to which systemic transphobia and ciscentrism are built into the healthcare system—from medical education to EMR and insurance billing. This, more so than individual instances of provider bias, has created the current state of population-level transgender healthcare inequality and limited mobility, both in terms of long distance travel to access care and in terms of limited mobility through clinics at the micromobility scale. Our direct care approach allows us to support individual transgender people while remaining aware of the systemic forces that impact individuals and communities. Because the Trans Buddy Program uses a direct care approach that is centered on an individual client's needs, we can support individual transgender patients as they navigate these systems, helping them to access the healthcare that is every person's right.

Acknowledgments

The author would like to acknowledge Kristen Eckstrand, MD, PhD, and Lauren Mitchell, MA, for their essential work cofounding, developing, and leading the Trans Buddy Program, as well as RJ Robles, BA, for their leadership in the continued success and growth of the Trans Buddy Program.

E. Kale Edmiston, PhD, is a neuroscience researcher from rural Ohio who cofounded the Trans Buddy Program in 2014. He has spoken at numerous conferences on transgender health and healthcare, including GLMA,

Philadelphia Trans Health, and the Civil Liberties and Public Policy Conference. From 2014 to 2015, he was the co-director of the Program for LGBTI Health at Vanderbilt University, where he focused on increasing access to primary and preventive healthcare for transgender people via clinician education and patient-centered public health research, and peer advocacy and outreach.

REFERENCES

Agee, Bonita S., Ellen Funkhouser, Jeffery M. Roseman, Hala Fawal, Scott D. Holmberg, and Sten H. Vermund. 2007. "Migration Patterns following HIV Diagnosis among Adults Residing in the Nonurban Deep South." *AIDS Care* 18(Suppl. 1): 51–58. doi:10.1080/09540120600839355.

Barth, Jay, and L. Martin Overby. 2003. "Are Gay Men and Lesbians in the South the New 'Threat'?: Regional Comparisons of the Contact Theory." *Politics & Policy* 31(3): 452–70.

Barton, B. 2010. "'Abomination'—Life as a Bible Belt Gay." *Journal of Homosexuality* 57(4): 465–84. doi:10.1080/00918361003608558.

Baunach, D. M., and E. O. Burgess. 2013. "Sexual Identity in the American Deep South: The Concordance and Discordance of Sexual Activity, Relationships, and Identities." *Journal of Homosexuality* 60(9): 1315–35.

Bradford, Judith, Sari L. Reisner, Julie A. Honnold, and Jessica Xavier. 2013. "Experiences of Transgender-Related Discrimination and Implications for Health: Results from the Virginia Transgender Health Initiative Study." *American Journal of Public Health* 103(10): 1820–9. doi:10.2105/AJPH/2012.300796.

Cahill, Sean, Robbie Singal, Chris Grasso, Dana King, Kenneth Mayer, Kellan Baker, and Harvey Makadon. 2014. "Do Ask, Do Tell: High Levels of Acceptability by Patients of Routine Collection of Sexual Orientation and Gender Identity Data in Four Diverse American Community Health Centers." *PLoS One* 9(9): e107104. doi:10.1371/journal.pone.0107104.

Carabez, Rebecca, Marion Pellegrini, Andrea Mankovitz, Mickey Eliason, and Megan Scott. 2015. "Does Your Organization Use Gender Inclusive Forms?: Nurses' Confusion about Trans* Terminology." *Journal of Clinical Nursing* 24(21/22): 3306–16. doi:10.1111/jocn.12942.

CDC (Centers for Disease Control and Prevention). 2013a. MMWR 2013;62 (Suppl 3):[9–104]

———. 2013b. "State-Specific Healthy Life Expectancy at Age 65 Years—United States, 2007–2009." *Morbidity and Mortality Weekly Report* 62(28): 561–66.

Conron, Kerith Jane, Scout, and S. Bryn Austin. 2008. "'Everyone Has a Right to, Like, Check Their Box': Findings on a Measure of Gender Identity from a Cognitive Testing Study with Adolescents." *Journal of LGBT Health Research* 4(1): 1–9. doi:10.1080/15574090802412572.

Cotton, Trystan. 2012. *Transgender Migrations: The Bodies, Borders, and Politics of Transition.* New York: Routledge.

Cruz, Taylor M. 2014. "Assessing Access to Care for Transgender and Gender Nonconforming People: A Consideration of Diversity in Combating Discrimination." *Social Science & Medicine* 110: 65–73. doi:10.1016/j.socscimed.2014.03.032.
Currah, Paisley, and Tara Mulqueen. 2011. "Securitizing Gender: Identity, Biometrics, and Transgender Bodies at the Airport." *Social Research* 78(2): 557–82.
DeNavas-Walt, Carmen, Bernadette D. Proctor, and Jessica C. Smith. 2011. *Income, Poverty and Health Insurance Coverage in the United States: 2010.* US Census Bureau, Current Population Reports, P60–239. Washington, DC: US Government Printing Office.
Edmiston E. Kale, Cameron A. Donald, Alice Rose Sattler, J. Klint Peebles, Jesse M. Ehrenfeld, and Kristen Laurel Eckstrand. 2016. "Opportunities and Gaps in Transgender Primary Healthcare: A Systematic Review." *Transgender Health* 1(1): 216–30. doi:10.1089/trgh.2016.0019.
Ellis, Dillon, Laura Panattoni, Amy Meehan, Judith Chuang, Caroline Wilson, and Ming Tai-Seale. 2015. "Using Unlicensed Health Coaches to Improve Care for Insured Patients with Diabetes and Hypertension: Patient and Physician Perspectives on Recruitment and Uptake." *Population Health Management.* 19(5): 332–40. doi:10.1089/pop.2015.0095.
Ellis, Mark, and Clara Muschkin. 1996. "Migration of Persons with AIDS—A Search for Support from Elderly Parents?" *Social Science & Medicine* 43(7): 1109–18. doi:10.1016/0277-9536(96)00031-7.
Finkler, Kaja, Cynthia Hunter, and Rick Iedema. 2008. "What Is Going On? Ethnography in Hospital Spaces." *Journal of Contemporary Ethnography* 37(2): 246–50. doi:10.1177/0891241607313398.
Grant, Jaime M., Lisa A. Mottet, Justin Tanis, Jack Harrison, Jody L. Herman, and Mara Keisling. 2011. *Injustice at Every Turn: A Report of the National Transgender Discrimination Survey.* Washington: National Center for Transgender Equality and National Gay and Lesbian Task Force.
Green, Jamison. 2014. "Transsexual Surgery May Be Covered by Medicare." *LGBT Health* 1(4): 256–58. doi:10.1089/lgbt.2014.0076.
Gutierrez, Andrea. 2008. "Geografia, Transporte, y Movilidad." *Espacios* 37: 100–7.
Hasenbush, Amira, Andrew R. Flores, Angeliki Kastanis, Brad Sears, and Gary J. Gates. 2014. "The LGBT Divide: A Data Portrait of the South, Midwest, and Mountain States." Williams Institute, UCLA School of Law.
Herman, Jody L., Christy Mallory, and Bianca D.M. Wilson. 2016. "Estimates of Transgender Populations in States with Legislation Impacting Transgender People." Williams Institute, UCLA School of Law.
Horvath, Keith J., Alex Iantaffi, Rebecca Swinburne-Romine, and Walter Bockting. 2014. "A Comparison of Mental Health, Substance Use, and Sexual Risk Behaviors between Rural and Non-Rural Transgender Persons." *Journal of Homosexuality* 61(8): 1117–30. doi:10.1080/00918369.2014.872502.
Human Rights Campaign and Trans People of Color Coalition. 2016. *Addressing Anti-transgender Violence: Exploring Realities, Challenges and Solutions.* Retrieved from https://assets2.hrc.org/files/assets/resources/HRC-AntiTransgenderViolence-0519.pdf.
Institute of Medicine (US) Committee on Lesbian, Gay, Bisexual, and Transgender Health Issues and Research Gaps and Opportunities. 2011. Washington, DC:

National Academies Press. Retrieved from https://www.ncbi.nlm.nih.gov/books/NBK64806/.

James-Abra, S., L. A. Tarasoff, d. green, R. Epstein, S. Anderson, S. Marvel, L. S. Steele, and L. E. Ross. 2015. "Trans People's Experiences with Assisted Reproduction Services: A Qualitative Study." *Human Reproduction* 30(6): 1365–74. doi:10.1093/humrep/dev087.

Jann, Jamieson T., E. Kale Edmiston, and Jesse M. Ehrenfeld. 2015. "Important Considerations for Addressing LGBT Health Care Competency." *American Journal of Public Health* 105(11): e8. doi:10.2105/AJPH.2015.302864.

Khalili, J., L. B. Leung, and A. L. Diamant. 2015. "Finding the Perfect Doctor: Identifying Lesbian, Gay, Bisexual, and Transgender-Competent Physicians." *American Journal of Public Health* 105(6): 1114–19. doi:10.2105/AJPH.2014.302448.

Lombardi, Emilio, R. A. Wilchins, D. Priesing, and Diane Malouf. 2001. "Gender Violence: Transgender Experiences with Violence and Discrimination." *Journal of Homosexuality* 42(1): 89–101.

Mananzala, Rickke, and Dean Spade. 2007. "The Non-Profit Industrial Complex and Trans Resistance." *Sexuality Research and Social Policy* 5(1): 53–71.

Mao, Liang, Jeanne-Marie R. Stacciarini, Rebekah Smith, and Brenda Wiens. 2015. "An Individual-Based Rurality Measure and Its Health Application: A Case Study of Latino Immigrants in North Florida, USA." *Social Science & Medicine* 147(2015): 300–8. doi:10.1016/j.socscimed.2015.10.064.

McCann, Edward. 2015. "People Who Are Transgender: Mental Health Concerns." *Journal of Psychiatric and Mental Health Nursing* 22(1): 76–81. doi:10.1111/jpm.12190.

McCann, Edward, and Danika Sharek. 2014. "Challenges to and Opportunities for Improving Mental Health Services for Lesbian, Gay, Bisexual, and Transgender People in Ireland: A Narrative Account." *International Journal of Mental Health Nursing* 23(6): 423–33. doi:10.1111/inm.12081.

Miller, Lisa R., and Eric Anthony Grollman. 2015. "The Social Costs of Gender Nonconformity for Transgender Adults: Implications for Discrimination and Health." *Sociological Forum* 30(3): 809–31. doi:10.111/socf.12193.

Poteat, Tonia, Danielle German, and Deanna Kerrigan. 2013. "Managing Uncertainty: A Grounding Theory of Stigma in Transgender Health Care Encounters." *Social Science & Medicine* 84: 22–29. doi:10.1016/j.socscimed.2013.02.019.

Roberts, Tiffany K., and Corinne R. Fantz. 2014. "Barriers to Quality Health Care for the Transgender Population." *Clinical Biochemistry* 47(10–11): 983–87. doi:10.1016/j.clinbiochem.2014.02.009.

Roche, Kirsten, and Corey Keith. 2014. "How Stigma Affects Healthcare Access for Transgender Sex Workers." *British Journal of Nursing* 23(21): 1147–52. doi:10.12968/bjon.2014.23.21.1147.

Roller, Cyndi Gale, Carol Sedlak, and Claire Burke Draucker. 2015. "Navigating the System: How Transgender Individuals Engage in Health Care Services." *Journal of Nursing Scholarship* 47(5): 417–24. doi:10.1111/jnu.12160.

Rosen, Dennis. 2014. *Vital Conversations: Improving Communication between Providers and Patients.* New York: Columbia University Press.

Safer, Joshua D., Eli Coleman, Jamie Feldman, Robert Garofalo, Wylie Hembree, Asa Radix, and Jae Sevelius. 2016. "Barriers to Healthcare for Transgender Individuals." *Current Opinions in Endocrinology Diabetes and Obesity* 23(2): 168–71. doi:10.1097/MED.0000000000000227.

Schrock, Douglas, Daphne Holden, and Lori Reid. 2004. "Creating Emotional Resonance: Interpersonal Emotion Work and Motivation Framing in a Transgender Community." *Social Problems* 51(1): 61–81.

Snelgrove John W., Amanda M. Jasudavisius, Bradley W. Rowe, Evan M. Head, and Greta R. Bauer. 2012. "'Completely Out-at-Sea' with 'Two-Gender Medicine': A Qualitative Analysis of Physician-Side Barriers to Providing Healthcare for Transgender Patients." *BMC Health Service Research* 12(1): 110. doi:10.1186/1472-6963-12-110.

Stotzer, Rebecca L. 2009. "Violence against Transgender People: A Review of the United States Data." *Aggression and Violent Behavior* 14: 170–9.

Tanser, Frank, Till Barnighausen, Alain Vandormael, and Adiran Dobra. 2015. "HIV Treatment Cascade in Migrants and Mobile Populations." *Current Opinion in HIV & AIDS* 10(6): 430–38.

Vindrola-Padros, Cecilia, and Ginger A. Johnson. 2015. "Children Seeking Health Care: International Perspectives on Children's Use of Mobility to Obtain Health Services." In *Movement, Mobilities, and Journeys, Geographies of Children and Young People,* ed. Caitriona Ni Laoire, Allen White, and Tracey Skelton, 289–306. Singapore: Springer.

White-Hughto, Jaclyn M., Sari L. Reisner, and John E. Pachankis. 2015. "Transgender Stigma and Health: A Critical Review of Stigma Determinants, Mechanisms, and Interventions." *Social Science & Medicine* 147: 222–31. doi:10.1016/j.socscimed.2015.11.010.

Wilson, Erin C., Yea-Hung Chen, Sean Arayasirikul, Conrad Wenzel, and H. Fisher Raymond. 2015. "Connecting the Dots: Examining Transgender Women's Utilization of Transition-Related Medical Care and Associations with Mental Health, Substance Use, and HIV." *Journal of Urban Health* 92(1): 182–92. doi:10.1007/s11524-014-9921-4.

Woodberry, Robert D., and Christian S. Smith. 1998. "Fundamentalism et al.: Conservative Protestants in America." *Annual Review of Sociology* 24: 25–26.

CHAPTER 10

Leading mHealth in Myanmar's Smartphone Revolution

Perrie Briskin and Sara Lucía Gallo

In 2010, Myanmar's military government started making political and economic concessions to open up the country after more than fifty years of international sanctions and isolation. At this time, due to tight government restrictions, a mobile phone SIM card from the government-owned telecom company cost around US$1,500 and less than 1 percent of the population had access to the Internet (Hindstrom 2016). Just four years later, foreign telecom competitors were admitted to the Myanmar market and, overnight, the price of a SIM card dropped to US$1.50. Following a landslide democratic election in November 2015 that brought iconic Nobel Peace Prize laureate Daw Aung San Suu Kyi to power, Myanmar is now considered the fastest-growing economy in the world (Myers 2016). Myanmar is changing at a rapid rate, and digital technology is a key driver of the country's momentum.

Population Services International (PSI), a global health nongovernmental organization (NGO), has worked in Myanmar since 1995. PSI uses social marketing to achieve positive health outcomes. Social marketing is a strategy that uses marketing concepts such as product design, appropriate pricing, sales and distribution, and communication to influence positive behaviors. PSI Myanmar's (PSI-M) social marketing programs distribute subsidized health products through commercial sector outlets like pharmacies and retailers. Moreover, PSI-M has a franchise of over 1,300 private general practitioners, who receive training and subsidized health commodities in exchange for quality health service delivery and data collection.

One of PSI-M's main pillars is reproductive health (RH) products and services to help women plan their families and thereby improve reproductive and maternal health. Historically, PSI-M has relied on traditional communication channels such as television, radio, interpersonal communicators, and information, education, and communication (IEC) materials to encourage behavior change. The recent digital revolution in Myanmar, however, has created a new realm of possibilities to reach target populations with information. This is a new form of "mobility" in Myanmar society whereby users are acquiring new knowledge, tools, and skills to advance economically and socially amidst rapid cultural change (Salazar 2010: 54).

In 2014, PSI-M launched "maymay," Myanmar's first maternal health mobile application (app), in partnership with one of the country's new foreign telecom companies and a local technology social enterprise firm. The maymay app has brought reproductive, maternal, and child health information to the fingertips of a much larger audience than could easily access health information prior to Myanmar's digital revolution. So far, maymay has returned very positive results. It remains the most-used mobile app for maternal health in Myanmar, with over forty thousand active users (defined as users who open the app at least once a month). Currently, a randomized control trial is evaluating maymay's impact and the extent to which its use can lead to improved maternal and child health outcomes.

As the digital landscape in Myanmar continues to evolve, PSI-M is poised to engage with rapid societal changes in order to deliver health messaging that enables positive behavior change. The purpose of this chapter is to highlight the technological changes in Myanmar as a form of mobility, where technology is producing tools and streamlining processes that are narrowing the gaps between the population's health information needs and wants and their fulfillment, thereby transforming the economic, social, and cultural landscape of the country by offering citizens new opportunities for upward mobility. Myanmar is an unusual case study because these changes are taking place in a very short period of time. The maymay app is one example of how technology is making much-needed and desired information accessible to large segments of the population through a medium that was previously unavailable.

The Need for Reproductive and Maternal Health Services

Myanmar is undergoing a remarkable transformation. Despite its imminent changes, decades of dictatorial rule and underinvestment have left the country underdeveloped, with a fragile health system and some of the worst health outcomes in the southeast Asia region. Maternal and neonatal conditions are at the top of Myanmar's national burden of disease list. The maternal mortality ratio has been reduced from 237 per 100,000 births in 2006 to 178 in 2015, but it remains one of the highest in the region, and progress has been sluggish in comparison to neighboring countries (World Bank 2015). As part of the 2014 National Strategic Plan to improve maternal and child health, the government of Myanmar has committed to provide proper antenatal care, promote skilled and institutional delivery of post-natal care, expand post-abortion care and access to quality birth spacing (contraception) products, strengthen adolescent reproductive health, streamline referral systems, and develop the capacity of community volunteers.

Reproductive health faces numerous challenges in Myanmar, particularly for sexually active and unmarried women. Myanmar remains a very traditional society with strong cultural and religious values placed on women's virginity and modesty. The government limits RH services to married women, which makes the private sector the main provider of RH services to young or unmarried women. Contraceptives are generally available, but can be difficult to obtain for low-income women, especially those in rural areas. Abortion is generally illegal and punishable by imprisonment. Yet, approximately 250,000 women get illegal abortions every year, making it among the leading causes of maternal mortality in the country (Shealy 2016). PSI-M has been working closely with the Myanmar Ministry of Health (MoH) for over twenty years to improve these reproductive and maternal health indicators. PSI-M conducts social marketing and behavior change campaigns to generate demand for RH products and services. In the last five years, PSI-M's network of over 1,300 private providers and close to 2,000 community workers has provided around eight million family-planning consultations.

Emergence of Digital Media in Myanmar

Before Myanmar started its transition to democracy, the military junta had imposed artificial caps on access to smartphones in order to limit communication. In 2010, when mobile phone SIM cards cost over US$1,500 and the average annual income was less than US$200, the state-owned Myanmar Post and Telecommunications (MPT) was the only mobile phone carrier (Motlagh 2014). As a result, in 2011, Myanmar had the second-lowest rate of mobile phone use per capita in the world, succeeded only by North Korea.

In 2013, the international telecom companies Telenor and Ooredoo were given licenses to provide mobile phone and Internet services. In 2014, both started selling SIM cards with a 3G connection for only US$1.50. As described by a student quoted in *Bloomberg News,* "We have been waiting so long for this—a lifetime. . . . Our country is finally coming out of the darkness. This will have a big impact on how we live and grow" (Motlagh 2014). The student was right; life in Myanmar has not been the same since.

After the drop in SIM card prices in 2014, mobile phone and Internet access has soared. Network towers have been built throughout the country, with 90 percent of the population reported to have Internet access as of March 2017 ("46m People in Myanmar" 2017). As of August 2016, Myanmar—a country of fifty-four million—had forty-five million active SIM card subscriptions, with an 80 percent smartphone usage rate (UN 2016; Cunningham 2016). This is remarkable considering that Africa's 2016 smartphone adoption rate is only 30 percent (GSMA 2016). Myanmar is embracing new technology faster than any other part of the developing world. As noted in the *Atlantic,* "there is a phrase repeated over and over again in Myanmar: From no power to solar, from no banks to digital currencies, from no computers and no Internet to capable smartphones with fast 3G connections. . . . There is little incumbency" (Mod 2016).

The quality of mobile and Internet signals remains spotty, but mobile phones have undoubtedly become a sign of social currency and upward mobility. Men and women prefer smartphones for using apps like Facebook and Viber. Touch phones are considered more "modern" and are directly associated with higher social status and financial independence, which is an aspiration for both men and women (Zainudeen and Galpaya 2015). The cost of smartphones is also continually dropping. In March 2016, Ooredoo launched a 30,000 MMK (US$24) smartphone (Trautwein 2016), and the secondhand smartphone market has also ballooned in the streets of downtown Yangon, Myanmar's largest city (Han 2016).

Another driver of smartphones' high adoption rate has been Myanmar's exceptionally high literacy rate. While Myanmar has over 135 ethnic groups, most with their own languages, the government's public schools teach only Burmese, the language of the dominant Burmese ethnic group (Michaels 2014). In 2016, the World Bank reported that 76 percent of the country's population was literate in Burmese ("Literacy Rate, Adult Total (% of People Ages 15 and above)" 2016). This high literacy rate enables the population to use apps like Facebook, Viber, and maymay with greater ease than countries with lower literacy rates.

Although Internet signals are expanding exponentially, actual access to the Internet via mobile phones varies greatly from urban to rural settings. According to a 2016 LIRNEasia survey (Galpaya and Zainudeen 2016), despite significant gains in recent years, rural mobile ownership rates continue to lag behind urban rates, at 53 percent to 79 percent. The urban-rural gap widens further when it comes to the ability to purchase a mobile phone (82 percent in urban areas versus 13 percent in rural), a SIM card (84 percent urban versus 22 percent rural), and mobile pay-as-you-go credit in their villages (96 percent in urban versus 60 percent in rural). The purposes of mobile phones are similar for both urban and rural populations, with the most common use being for social purposes followed by livelihood. However, people with higher incomes perceive greater benefits than people with lower incomes in terms of improvement of their economic status, level of knowledge and skills, social relationships, and happiness when owning a smartphone (Galpaya 2015).

How Women Interact with Digital Media

In Myanmar, barriers to mobile phone access are marked more strongly by economic limitations than by gender factors. Although traditional cultural norms continue to ascribe women and men different societal roles, where men are expected to be breadwinners and women the masters of household matters, a recent study has shown that the main barrier for female mobile phone ownership in Myanmar is actually affordability and school or work outside the home. Men were unsurprisingly given priority as they are more likely to work outside the house. Nonetheless, respondents did not express opposition to women owning a phone. Inaccessibility was more a matter of being unable to pay for multiple mobile phones in one household (Zainudeen and Galpaya 2015). In cases where women worked or studied outside the home, they were given priority for mobile phone ownership. The study noted that in fact women play an active role in deciding whether to buy a mobile phone as they usually manage household finances.

Women in Myanmar are 20 percent less likely than men to own a mobile phone, and the gender gap is even greater among lower-income households (Galpaya and Zainudeen 2016). However, as the economy and labor market expand, women are taking more work opportunities outside the home, sometimes even migrating to more urban areas. These changes are increasingly giving women greater purchasing and negotiating power around mobile phone ownership.

Myanmar's Technological Advances as a Form of Mobility

As sociocultural anthropologist Noel B. Salazar (2010) explains, mobility is not just geographic or physical but also entails the mobility of cultures. Citing Ziegler and Schwanen, Salazar (2017: 1) describes mobility as the ability to overcome "any type of distance between a here and a there, which can be situated in physical, electronic, social, psychological or other kinds of space." In Myanmar, technological advancements go hand in hand with the political and economic changes the country is undergoing, thereby cultivating a culture of mobility represented by a growing labor market, increasing disposable income, migration to urban areas, and embrace of foreign culture. Mobile phones, particularly smartphones, are a mobility tool that expands people's access to information and opportunities. According to an International Growth Centre (2016) study, Yangon's GDP growth is expected to be one of the highest globally between 2012 and 2030, with accelerated foreign direct investment creating new opportunities. International brands such as Coca-Cola and Kentucky Fried Chicken received outstanding acceptance upon their arrival in the country in 2012 and 2015, respectively. Moreover, mobile phone access to "modern" influences such as fashion, celebrity lifestyles, and dating practices are challenging traditional gender norms (Zainudeen and Galpaya 2015). Notwithstanding, these advancements further highlight the inequalities among those who embrace these changes and those who cannot. For organizations such as PSI looking to support populations most in need—who may or may not be able to afford mobile phones—it is important to understand the limits of digital technology in order to prevent falling into ineffective one-size-fits-all solutions.

Maymay Mobile App

Maymay is Myanmar's first-ever maternal and child health Android app. As of May 2016, maymay has been downloaded over fifty thousand times and transferred offline via Bluetooth peer-to-peer file-sharing app Zapya over thirty thousand times. Forty thousand users (50 percent) are active, meaning they open the app at least once a month. This is impressive in comparison to estimates that the average app downloaded from the Google Play Store loses over 75 percent of its users within just the first few months (Chen 2015). As mentioned before, Myanmar has some of the worst maternal and child health outcomes in the region. Therefore, maymay's goal is simple: by delivering fun and easy-to-understand information directly to smartphones, maymay can help Myanmar mothers take better care of their babies and themselves and therefore lead healthier lives.

Maymay Is Conceived

Maymay was made possible by a partnership between Ooredoo, an international telecom company; PSI-M; and Koe Koe Tech, a local technology social enterprise firm. In 2014, Ooredoo received an mWomen grant from the

Groupe Spécial Mobile Association (GSMA) to build an app for women. It was upon receiving this grant that Ooredoo approached PSI-M and Koe Koe Tech with the idea of creating an Android app for moms using short message service (SMS) text messages that had already been created by the Mobile Alliance for Maternal Action (MAMA), an organization dedicated to delivering health messages to new mothers via mobile phone.

Maymay was the product of a collaborative approach among the three partners: Ooredoo, PSI-M, and Koe Koe Tech. Ooredoo acted as the donor, in partnership with GSMA, and conducted initial post-launch assessment of the app to measure user acceptability. PSI-M translated and adapted MAMA content for Myanmar, navigated the MoH approval process (required for all PSI-M communication materials), and coordinated focus groups with key audiences to inform the app's development. Lastly, Koe Koe Tech served as not only the technology and design lead, but also the owner of maymay. From its inception, maymay's long-term sustainability plan was based on Koe Koe Tech owning the app and making it sustainable through in-app advertising. As a nimble start-up, Koe Koe Tech could theoretically keep the app more current than if it were managed by a large organization like PSI-M or Ooredoo.

The MAMA content provided an initial roadmap that guided the early stages of development. From 2011 to 2015, MAMA licensed several maternal and child health SMS messages at no cost to organizations around the world. MAMA messages were designed to be delivered as text messages to phones three times a week, from week five of pregnancy to the child's third birthday. The SMS maternal health messages were simple—for example, "Make a plan with your family to put your new baby to the breast in the first hour. Your creamy first milk will protect him from illness." By the time maymay adapted MAMA messages in 2014, the messages had already been shown to have a positive impact in places like Bangladesh and South Africa ("MAMA Bangladesh (Aponjon) Formative Research Report" 2013).

One of the first steps in developing maymay was to have the app be informed by key Myanmar audiences, including mothers, fathers, and midwives. PSI-M conducted a series of focus groups with these audiences in the summer of 2014. Focus group participants were asked where they usually got health information and what suggestions they had for making the Burmese translation of MAMA messages easier to understand. Additionally, focus group participants were observed logging in and exploring an early prototype of the app. These groups provided crucial feedback that led to significant changes in the app interface to make it easier for the low tech literacy of Myanmar audiences by, for example, changing user login requirements.

Maymay Is Born

In September 2014, maymay softly launched in the Google Play Store. A pregnant local celebrity was recruited to be maymay's champion and promoter. A maymay Facebook page was created and boosted using Facebook Ads to promote the app. Fans used the maymay Facebook page to learn more about the app and submit their questions and comments.

One of maymay's greatest challenges was obtaining MoH approval. In Myanmar, all health communication materials require MoH approval before public release or risk removal. Maymay was finally approved by MoH in March 2015, ten months after being submitted for review. This was a tremendous feat as it was the first mobile app ever to receive any kind of approval from MoH.[1]

In the first year of its launch, maymay was downloaded over ten thousand times. However, significant challenges kept it from achieving even greater uptake. The first difficulty was miscalculations in the distribution strategy. At the request of Ooredoo, maymay was initially made exclusive to Ooredoo customers. This exclusivity clause was hard to communicate to

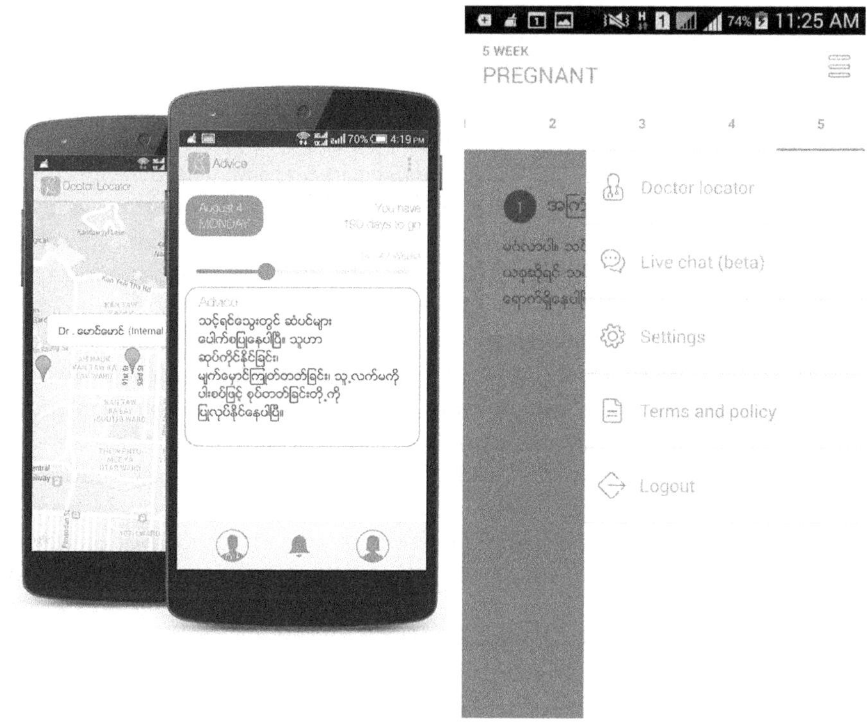

Figure 10.1 Screenshots of maymay 1.0, released in September 2014. Image courtesy of Koe Koe Tech Co., Ltd.

customers and limited the impact of maymay's mission—to improve maternal and child health in Myanmar.

The second challenge was the likability of the app itself. While the MAMA messages provided crucial content and initial app structure, passive one-way messages were not enough to keep maymay users engaged. Moreover, while the app was in some ways simple to use, user feedback revealed that it was not optimized for an audience that was using apps for the very first time. People were not familiar with logging in to an app using their phone number.[2] Likewise, most people in Myanmar are unfamiliar with maps, whether digital or paper, which made the map-based Doctor Locator feature confusing for users. To address these challenges, in the fall of 2015—one year after launch—Ooredoo, Koe Koe Tech, and PSI-M gave maymay a transformative facelift. And thus, maymay 2.0 was born.

Maymay Is Reborn

Maymay 2.0 was released in January 2016 with significant changes made to almost every aspect of the app, including interface, content, and distribution. The changes came from a rapid prototyping strategy adopted by Koe Koe Tech, which consisted of producing an early iteration of the product and testing it with users on an ongoing basis. Koe Koe Tech staff visited a Yangon public park or market once a week and asked strangers to use the maymay app for up to five minutes with no instructions. This was meant to model how the maymay app would be used in real life. The demographics were varied—from young, unmarried men and women to mothers and fathers. Koe Koe Tech observed how each user experienced maymay, including any barriers to use and which features attracted the most attention.

Rapid prototyping quickly exposed a barrage of usability issues. Some functions perceived as easy by the app's developers proved to be not intuitive for users, which quickly reduced interest in the app. Some users would quit the app within only one to three minutes. The most common problems included logging in, navigating through the different menu options that contained English words, and finding doctor contact information. If these problems were encountered in the city of Yangon, the most tech-savvy of settings, the user dropoff would be even greater in less developed areas.

With these findings, PSI-M and Koe Koe Tech set off to simplify the app. Now, upon opening maymay 2.0, users can see all the menu options at once with no login required. Only after using the app a few times will users be asked to sign into maymay with their mobile number. Moreover, words and numbers in English were replaced with 100 percent Burmese text and numbers. The Doctor Locator map was also transformed into a list that users can sort by townships and that shows basic information such as the working hours and phone numbers of PSI-M's clinics.

The next challenge was revising the maymay content. Facebook fans and rapid prototyping participants indicated that users craved more interaction than the basic, one-way message notifications. PSI-M and Koe Koe Tech looked closely at other learning apps, such as the popular language app Duolingo, and thought the same gamified model could be applied to maymay. Consequently, PSI-M transformed the MAMA messages into hundreds of multiple-choice questions, where users answer a set of questions for each week of their pregnancy. For every question answered correctly, users receive points. Moreover, PSI-M engaged technical experts such as nutritionists, obstetricians, and gynecologists on a temporary basis to develop longer content on popular subjects such as neonatal care, breastfeeding, and child nutrition.

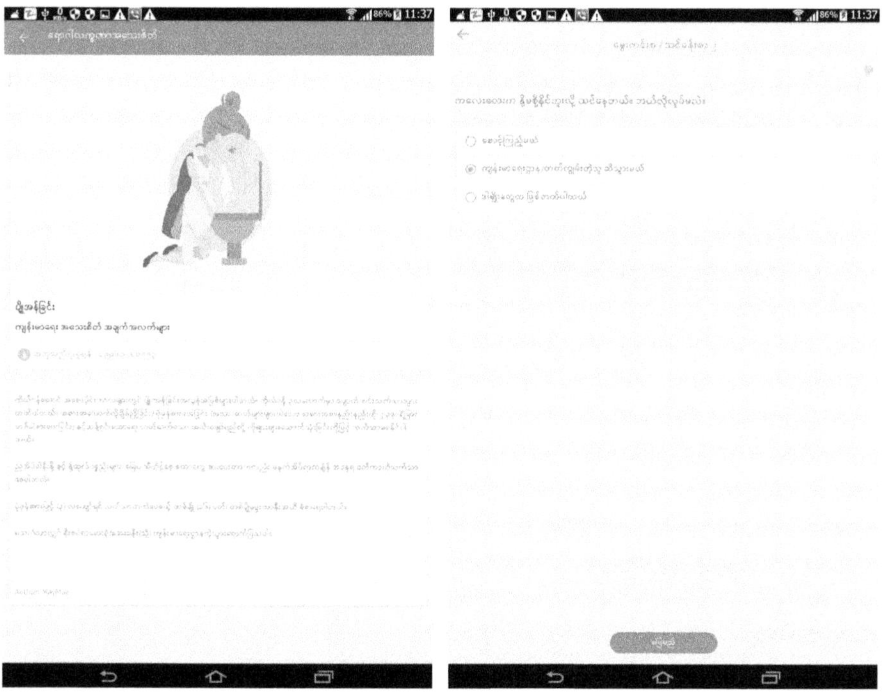

Figure 10.2 Screenshots of maymay 2.0, released January 2016. This version added quizzes and articles to engage users. Screenshot courtesy of Koe Koe Tech Co., Ltd.

Screenshot 1: "Nausea and Vomiting During Pregnancy"
The article includes information about how to manage morning sickness (nausea) and at what point women should see a doctor.

Screenshot 2: Newborn / Lesson 2
When breastfeeding, my baby does not seem to suck well. What should I do?
Wait and see.
Go and see your health care provider [Answer].
This is very common, no need to take any action.

In 2017, the maymay interface was updated to more closely mirror Facebook's scrolling newsfeed. As one of Koe Koe Tech's developers put it, "Because of Facebook, people in Myanmar prefer to scroll, not tap."

Moreover, PSI-M and Koe Koe Tech also pushed to change the distribution model for maymay. The exclusivity clause was detrimental to increasing the app's user base. A compromise was struck with Ooredoo: maymay would be made available to users from all mobile carriers, but Ooredoo banner ads would display in the app for non-Ooredoo users. Furthermore, user insights showed that most Myanmar users do not have email addresses or credit cards and, by extension, did not have a Google Play account, thereby making it impossible to download maymay from the Google Play Store. This inability to access maymay through Google Play has continued to be a problem because no alternative app store exists.

To address the lack of email addresses, Koe Koe Tech created a "Use App" link on the maymay Facebook page that connects directly to a splash page on Koe Koe Tech's website, where users can download the app Android package kit (APK) file. While downloading the APK is a cumbersome experience, forcing users to manually open the application from

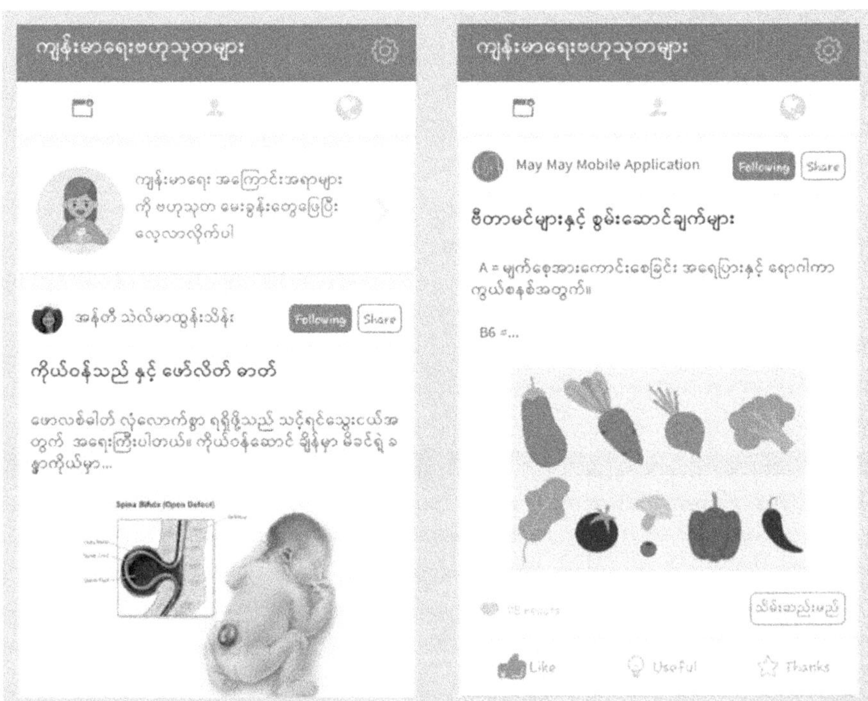

Figure 10.3 Screenshots of maymay update released in 2017. App now includes a Facebook-style newsfeed for users to scroll through. Screenshot courtesy of Koe Koe Tech Co., Ltd.

their phone's data files, Myanmar mobile users are more familiar with this process than with downloading from an app store. Koe Koe Tech has also set up a referral incentive feature whereby people can earn a small reward (e.g., 200 MMK, or US$0.17) for sharing maymay via the Bluetooth peer-to-peer file-sharing app Zapya, the most common app distribution channel in Myanmar. In 2017, maymay was transferred via Zapya to over thirty thousand new phones. Although this is more convenient for users, it comes at a high cost for Koe Koe Tech and PSI: it is not possible to glean app-usage data from users who have downloaded the app offline via Bluetooth and proceed to use the app entirely offline. The value of maymay to the user is its easy-to-understand maternal health information, which maymay accomplishes regardless. However, offline transfers of the app make it difficult for Koe Koe Tech and PSI to measure its impact.

Users have responded very favorably to the app's changes. Maymay 2.0 was downloaded over fifty thousand times in its first nine months, compared to just ten thousand times for maymay 1.0 in its first year. The new multiple-choice quizzes are by far the most popular aspect of the app and the maymay Facebook page continues to be extremely popular—it now boasts over 170,000 fans. The Facebook page has created a helpful feedback loop where the most commonly asked questions submitted on the Facebook page eventually become articles and multiple-choice questions in the maymay app.

Maymay's Check-up

Maymay's main goal has always been educating mothers and caretakers of children to adopt healthy behaviors that lead to better maternal and child health outcomes. New content continues to be created on an ongoing basis. To measure whether the application is in fact reaching this goal, in December 2014, Ooredoo conducted a telephone survey with 257 maymay users. Sixty-nine percent of respondents said that the app added value to their lives and 87 percent of respondents said they would recommend maymay to others.

To measure impact with a more robust methodology, in 2018, research partners will start a randomized control trial with 1,200 pregnant women, tracking their use of maymay and its impact on behavior change.[3] The study results should be available in late 2018. The study seeks to understand whether using the maymay app leads to behavior change, such as breastfeeding exclusively for the first six months and attending antenatal care visits. In the meantime, other studies conducted recently in Myanmar have shown the effectiveness of mobile SMS messages in the promotion of exclusive breastfeeding (Hmone 2017).

Moreover, user activity on maymay is closely monitored. A major advantage of an app, as opposed to an SMS service, is the user data collected—assuming the user connects to a data network at some point while using the app. The number of users, how often they open the app, what content is clicked on the most, and for how long—these are all key performance indicators (KPIs) that Koe Koe Tech regularly reports to PSI-M and that inform future app development. The app and the Facebook page provide a constant feedback loop, especially for content.

The maymay App in the Global mHealth Context

The maymay app joins hundreds of other projects around the world under the mHealth umbrella.[4] No definitive number of mHealth projects exists, but GSMA's Mobile for Development Trackers, a directory of mobile for development projects, lists over 1,200 mHealth projects ("mHealth Deployment Tracker" 2017). Such projects range from telephone hotlines to patient education tools (like maymay) to frontline health worker applications to electronic medical records. In terms of facilitating upward mobility, mHealth is especially enticing for NGOs and governments in low-income settings. While it does take resources to develop, a digital intervention can be simpler and more affordable than, for example, building new infrastructure or implementing new government policies.

The Importance of Measurement and Evaluation

One of the biggest critiques of mHealth is the lack of evaluation for impact and effectiveness. The WHO conducted a survey in 2011 that found only 12 percent of member states reported evaluating mHealth services (WHO 2011: 71). In 2015, researchers conducting a survey of sixty-nine mHealth projects across twenty-nine countries found that "while mHealth initiatives are being adopted by a wide range of health programs in low-, middle- and high-income countries, for a wide variety of purposes, evaluation of the health impact of these initiatives is either missing or weak" (Mookherji et al. 2015: 1228). Quality measurement and evaluation can, admittedly, be challenging across all areas of development. For mHealth, it is made all the more challenging by the rapid pace of technology, which often does not allow time for rigorous evaluation (MHTF 2014).

To address this gap between implementation and evaluation, in 2016 the WHO mHealth Technical Evidence Review Group released an mHealth evidence and reporting assessment (mERA) checklist (WHO 2016). This mERA checklist is meant to act as a guide for reporting on the effectiveness of mHealth services. It is a useful starting point and answers the call to create mHealth standards that optimize resources and prevent the duplication of products. The team behind maymay's randomized control trial that is currently underway has reviewed the mERA checklist and will address its sixteen items.

Mobility Study Methodologies

For mobility studies, mobile technology is a rare arena to target because it is not necessarily linked to physical movement. Nonetheless, as explained before, mobile phone use has totally changed Myanmar's social and economic landscape. As new forms of mobility emerge, and as they become more studied, methodologies too are being adapted. As Salazar (2017: 7) notes, some of the most frequently used methodologies for studying mobility, such as single-site visits, "no longer feel adequate for the realities of an increasingly mobile, shifting and interconnect world."

Mobile technology data on user behavior can be very powerful. This is why social and digital media advertising has been so successful at impacting people's behavior on- and offline, as seen in the impact of Facebook on political events in both the United States and Myanmar in recent years (Clark 2017). When it comes to the maymay app, programmers can easily follow users and observe their reactions in real time. In addition to the in-person focus groups and pre-testing prototypes with potential users, maymay used a specific set of key performance indicators—age, location, time spent, favorite maternal health topic areas, time of login, etc.—to finetune the future content and format of the app. These KPIs have become a treasure trove of data for Koe Koe Tech and its partners to ensure that the app is delivering on its objective.

The study of mobile technology as a form of mobility offers a stark contrast to traditional methods for "following" target populations. When studying the impact of mobile technology, there is typically an overabundance of data about the people who adopt this form of mobility, and those without mobile phones are at risk of being overlooked by researchers. The perils of a digital divide are another area of study altogether. Where mobile users easily and sometimes unknowingly convey data about their likes and dislikes, location, language, and attention span, non-users have no way of communicating with programmers, which presents a major challenge for mHealth interventions in poorer communities. As Salazar (2017: 14) adeptly argued, "mobility remains formidably difficult for many; sometimes more so than before. To understand mobility, we thus need to pay close attention also to immobility, to the structures . . . that facilitate certain movements and impede others."

The maymay app foresaw this challenge, and its developers were committed to translating the app to different ethnic languages in Myanmar. Moreover, PSI-M and Koe Koe Tech are focused on expanding maymay to more rural areas. Now that the country's most populous areas are covered by Internet networks, telecommunication companies are increasingly focused on expansion into rural areas (Hammond 2016). As Internet connectivity continues to increase, and as more people, especially in rural communities, purchase affordable smartphones, maymay will also continue to grow. However, that still does not resolve the purchasing-power gap between those who can afford a phone and connectivity and those who cannot, nor does it address the many other structural and economic barriers to accessing healthcare in general.

Reaching Populations Most in Need

mHealth projects in low-income countries are often criticized for their inability to reach those populations most in need—often those living in rural areas with scarce resources and little mobile network access. As is noted in a 2015 article about mobile phone penetration in Sub-Saharan Africa, "it is in impoverished rural areas, where the need to overcome healthcare barriers is greatest, that the reach of 'informal mhealth' has (so far) been most limited. Digital technologies tend to map onto existing (often deeply-rooted) social inequalities which become re-configured but not erased" (Hampshire et al. 2015, 98). While technology enables a mobility of culture, it cannot be implemented in a vacuum that ignores other barriers. For example, maymay can recommend that women give birth in a facility instead of at home, but maymay cannot ensure that a well-equipped facility is affordable, within reach, and actually safer for all mothers. New technology has to be embraced to reach wider audiences but it cannot transcend the complex web of barriers to other forms of mobility.

PSI-M's Top Five Learnings from the maymay App

In late 2015, the partnership with Ooredoo ended, but maymay continues to be owned by Koe Koe Tech and supported by PSI-M, both of which have dedicated staff on the project. Maymay will continue to be successful to the extent that it is regularly updated with new information targeted to users' needs and preferences, in terms of both content and ease of navigation. PSI-M has gathered the following five learnings for digital media project managers working in low-income settings:

1. Collaborate. Do not reinvent the wheel

With so many mHealth projects already created across the globe, there is great opportunity for collaboration between implementers. Whether it is with content, distribution, promotion, or app architecture, organizations can first explore partnerships instead of spending intensive resources creating brand-new platforms. For maymay, PSI-M was grateful to license the MAMA messages that kicked off the first version of the maymay app. In December 2015, however, the MAMA organization shuttered its doors. While the original messages are still available for download on its website, MAMA will unfortunately no longer be creating new, shareable, free content.[5]

There is also great potential for project managers to use popular platforms like Facebook to reach audiences rather than creating new channels from scratch. This allows for optimization of resources and enables users to continue accessing key information via channels they are already familiar with and prefer. With so many mHealth projects already being tested or implemented, it is becoming increasingly burdensome to start completely new projects. In Uganda, for instance, the government placed a moratorium on all mHealth projects, citing that a glut of digital health projects was distracting resources from areas of greater need (MHTF 2014). GSMA and Johns Hopkins University's Global mHeath Initiative are two examples of organizations attempting to connect and encourage collaboration between mHealth implementers.[6] The logistics around sharing (e.g., distribution of labor, licensing agreements, and translation) can be a challenge, but collaboration still takes fewer resources than starting from scratch. PSI-M is in conversation with other PSI country programs to adapt maymay for other contexts.

2. Make it user-focused

For mHealth projects to achieve impact, enable mobility, and sustain success, there are a myriad different aspects of the user experience to consider. The biggest lesson for maymay has been to make users the top priority. Initial user focus groups were conducted in conference rooms. Although useful, these focus groups did not accurately recreate the real user experience of maymay. It was only with rapid prototyping—asking people in public spaces to engage with maymay without any instructions—that PSI-M and Koe Koe Tech were able to understand the nuances of and barriers to users' experiences.

This lesson also applies to marketing and distribution. For maymay, different strategies have to be considered as the app expands into rural areas. In an environment where apps are shared over a Bluetooth connection and not downloaded from an app store, PSI-M and Koe Koe Tech have had to work to devise a distribution strategy to meet users where they already are. This has led to investment in promoting maymay in rural areas via Zapya transfer.

Another important user consideration is language and literacy. PSI-M and Koe Koe Tech have considered translating maymay into other ethnic languages. However, as previously mentioned, Myanmar has a very high literacy rate in Burmese. PSI-M and Koe Koe Tech have found that if a community reads more than one language, they often read Burmese as well as or better than their ethnic language. Understandably, this may not be an option in other contexts, where multiple languages, either in written or audio form, may have to be considered.

3. Commit to a long-term relationship with digital media

Embarking on a digital intervention is just the initial investment. In order to reap the long-term benefits, project managers need to commit continuous resources to pilot ideas, fix bugs, create content, interpret user data, and apply learnings. Just because an app is easy and quick for users to consume does not mean it is as easy and quick to create. Project managers need to budget resources that include quantitative and qualitative assessment of user engagement, including staff to make corresponding updates for the entire lifespan of the app.

4. Engage with local partners

One of the most rewarding aspects of the maymay app has been the relationship PSI-M has formed with Koe Koe Tech. PSI-M has the health expertise and solidity of an international organization, whereas Koe Koe Tech has the technical expertise plus the nimbleness of a start-up. Both organizations have been able to promote maymay and the partnership to attract additional funding opportunities.

Maymay has also been positively featured by National Public Radio (Leatherby 2015), National Geographic (Banks 2015), and all major local Myanmar news outlets (Myat 2014; Trautwein 2014). An article on *Mashable Asia* listed maymay as one of the eight apps revolutionizing maternal healthcare in developing nations (Dupere 2016). Moreover, the cofounders of Koe Koe Tech have personally introduced the app at high-profile international forums and conferences such as F8 (Facebook's Developer Conference), Women Deliver, and the Skoll World Forum. The app's success has undoubtedly been a result of the mix of the partners' expertise, respective competitive advantages, and commitment to working through challenges together. To solidify that commitment, PSI-M and Koe Koe Tech have entered into a multiyear teaming agreement to continue to work on mHealth projects together.[7]

5. Embrace new technology

Information communication technology is constantly changing. Sectors from health to news to entertainment have little choice but to adapt. For an organization like PSI-M, which has spent upwards of twenty years creating health pamphlets and television commercials, diving into a mobile app was uncharted territory. However, PSI-M's audiences were already making the transition to access all types of information through mobile phones and Facebook, so PSI-M could not miss the opportunity to meet them in their preferred spaces, even if it meant learning on the go.

Conclusion

Myanmar's transition to democracy, and its subsequent economic and digital transformations, are enabling upward mobility at an accelerated pace. People now have more access to information and income opportunities, which in turn is enabling higher levels of education, migration, and technology use. Smartphones are a mobility tool. Despite its limitations reaching Myanmar's poorest citizens, smartphones are revolutionizing Myanmar as they enable people to pursue what they want, whether it be friends, health information, news, or job and educational opportunities. For organizations looking to capitalize on vibrant digital markets, the learning curve is steep, especially in a country like Myanmar, which is quickly transitioning from zero Internet coverage to the widespread availability (and popularity) of smartphones. Digital media has the advantage of making users your friends, fans, followers, and subscribers, allowing implementers to get to know their users more intimately than ever before. Digital health initiatives should therefore closely follow their users' interests and preferences; they can inform product design and thereby ensure that messages remain relevant and that target populations remain tuned in.

Behavior change will never be a hard science. The more open, engaging, and receptive project managers are to their target audiences, the more likely their projects are to connect with their audiences and instill the intended change. The goal with maymay has always been to improve maternal and child health outcomes in Myanmar. While the aim is ambitious and overwhelming, considering Myanmar's current context, PSI-M and Koe Koe Tech will continue to strive toward creating measurable behavior change. This will be undertaken by continuing to listen to maymay users and creating health information that it is actionable, compelling, and (hopefully) a little bit fun.

Perrie Briskin is a digital project manager with a focus on health data and communication. At Population Services International (PSI) Myanmar, she led the strategy and development of digital information systems, social media campaigns, and mobile apps. She guides teams across private, public, and development sectors, forging unique partnerships. Prior to PSI, Briskin worked with the US government managing online health communication tools. She is passionate about user-centered design, a data-driven approach, and collaboration between organizations within the global digital health space.

Sara Lucía Gallo is from Colombia and moved to the United States in 2000. She completed her bachelor's degree in international affairs at Northeastern University and her master's degree in the same field at the Graduate Institute of International and Development Studies in Geneva, Switzerland. Following her master's degree, Gallo worked at Population Services International (PSI), first as a program coordinator for Latin America and the Caribbean, and later as a program manager for PSI Myanmar. Sara is passionate about reproductive health and currently works for Planned Parenthood Global, Latin America Region.

NOTES

1. The approval period took longer than expected because maymay was a new kind of communication tool for the MoH to review. PSI-M had to submit printed maymay content along with screenshots from the app.
2. Maymay users are required to enter their phone number as a way to set up their maymay account. It is important for measurement and evaluation purposes that unique maymay users be tracked. Entering a phone number, as opposed to a username and password, seemed the easiest way for maymay users to create accounts.
3. The randomized control trial will be conducted by Innovations for Poverty Action, the International Growth Centre, and economists at the University of Sydney and University of California Los Angeles, in partnership with Koe Koe Tech.
4. mHealth is defined by the World Health Organization as "medical and public health practice supported by mobile devices, such as mobile phones, patient monitoring devices, personal digital assistants (PDAs), and other wireless devices" (WHO 2011: 6).
5. Access the MAMA messages at: http://www.unfoundation.org/what-we-do/issues/global-health/mobile-health-for-development/mama.html.
6. Read more at the Global mHealth Initiative website (http://www.jhumhealth.org).

7. Whenever possible, PSI-M and Koe Koe Tech are committed to using open-sourced software and adapting content already created by other organizations willing to partner.

REFERENCES

"46m People in Myanmar Now Use the Internet, Up 10m from Last Year." 2017. *Coconuts Yangon,* 29 March. Retrieved 7 November 2017 from https://coconuts.co/yangon/news/ministry-of-communications-report-10-million-increase-in-internet-users-within-last-year/.

Banks, Ken. 2015. "How Smartphones Fill the Healthcare Gap in Myanmar." *National Geographic Blog,* 22 September. Retrieved 31 August 2016 from http://voices.nationalgeographic.com/2015/09/22/how-smartphones-fill-the-healthcare-gap-in-myanmar.

Chen, Andrew. 2015. "New Data Shows Losing 80% of Mobile Users Is Normal, and Why the Best Apps Do Better." *@andrewchen* (blog), 9 June. Retrieved 31 August 2016 from http://andrewchen.co/new-data-shows-why-losing-80-of-your-mobile-users-is-normal-and-that-the-best-apps-do-much-better/.

Clark, Doug Bock. 2017. "Myanmar's Internet Disrupted Society—And Fueled Extremists." *Wired,* 28 September. Retrieved 7 November 2017 from https://www.wired.com/story/myanmar-internet-disrupted-society-extremism/.

Cunningham, Susan. 2016. "Myanmar: 45 Million Mobile Phones and the $19 3G Smartphone." *Forbes Asia,* 10 August. Retrieved 7 November 2017 from https://www.forbes.com/sites/susancunningham/2016/08/10/myanmar-45-million-mobile-phones-and-the-19-3g-smartphone.

Dupere, Katie. 2016. "8 Apps Revolutionizing Maternal Health Care in Developing Nations." *Mashable Asia,* 13 March. Retrieved 31 August 2016 from http://mashable.com/2016/03/13/apps-maternal-health/#cD9ovRzrkOqJ.

Galpaya, Helani. 2015. "Knowledge, Information and Communication Habits and Needs in Myanmar: Stories from the Field." LIRNEasia and You can do it. Slide 30. Retrieved 31 August 2016 from http://lirneasia.net/wp-content/uploads/2015/08/2015-07-MyanmarBaselineSurveyICTuse-v9-1.pdf.

Galpaya, Helani and Ayesha Zainudeen. 2016. "Mobile Phones, Internet, Information, and Knowledge: Myanmar 2016." LIRNEasia and You can do it. Slide 55-65. Retrieved 7 November 2017 from http://lirneasia.net/wp-content/uploads/2017/09/Mobile-phones-Internet-information-and-knowledge-Myanmar-2016.pdf.

GSMA. 2016. *The Mobile Economy: Africa 2016.* London: GSMA. Retrieved 7 October 2017 from https://www.gsmaintelligence.com/research/?file=3bc21ea879a5b217b64d62fa24c55bdf&download.

Hammond, Clare. 2016. "Telenor Racks Up 14 Million Users." *Myanmar Times,* 11 February. Retrieved 31 August 2016 from http://www.mmtimes.com/index.php/business/technology/18928-telenor-racks-up-14-million-users.html.

Hampshire, Kate, Gina Portera, Samuel Asiedu Owusub, Simon Mariwahc, Albert Abanec, Elsbeth Robsond, Alister Munthalie, et al. 2015. "Informal m-Health: How

Are Young People Using Mobile Phones to Bridge Healthcare Gaps in Sub-Saharan Africa?" *Social Science & Medicine* 142: 90–99.

Han, Thi Ri. 2016. "Telecoms Boom Fuels Fierce Competition in Used Phone Market." *Frontier Myanmar,* 30 August. Retrieved 30 October 2016 from http://frontiermyanmar.net/en/telecoms-boom-fuels-fierce-competition-in-used-phone-market.

Hindstrom, Hanna. 2016. "The Perils of Burma's Internet Craze." *Foreign Policy,* 1 April. Retrieved 31 August 2016 from https://foreignpolicy.com/2016/04/01/the-perils-of-burmas-Internet-craze/.

Hmone, Myat Pan, Mu Li, Kingsley Agho, and Michael J. Dibley. 2017. "Impact of SMS Text Messages to Improve Exclusive Breastfeeding: A Randomized Controlled Trial in Myanmar." *FASEB Journal* 31(Suppl. 1). Retrieved 20 November 2017 from http://www.fasebj.org/content/31/1_Supplement/313.3.

International Growth Centre. 2016. "Yangon Urban Growth Analytics: A Comparative Information Base for Strategic Spatial Development in Yangon, Myanmar." *LSE Cities.* July 2016. Reference number C-53304-MYA-1. Retrieved 3 November 2016 from https://www.theigc.org/project/yangon-urban-growth-analytics/#outputs.

Leatherby, Lauren. 2015. "Smartphones Bring Happiness and Headaches to Myanmar." *Goats and Soda* (blog), Northwest Public Broadcasting, 14 September. Retrieved 31 August 2016 from http://www.npr.org/sections/goatsandsoda/2015/09/14/424701548/smartphones-bring-happiness-and-headaches-to-myanmar.

"MAMA Bangladesh (Aponjon) Formative Research Report." 2013. Mobile Alliance for Maternal Action. Retrieved 30 March 2018 from http://www.mhealthknowledge.org/resources/mama-bangladesh-aponjon-formative-research-report-0.

"mHealth Deployment Tracker." 2017. GSMA. Retrieved 7 November 2017 from https://www.gsma.com/mobilefordevelopment/m4d-tracker/mhealth-deployment-tracker/.

MHTF (Maternal Health Task Force). 2014. "mHealth for Maternal Health: mHealth Pilotitis – Time for Recovery or Relapse?" *MHTF Blog,* 31 March. Retrieved 31 August 2016 from https://www.mhtf.org/2014/03/31/mhealth-for-maternal-health-mhealth-pilotitis-time-for-recovery-or-relapse/.

Michaels, Samantha. 2014. "Pan-Ethnic Network Launches to Promote Multilingual Education in Burma." *The Irrawaddy,* 21 February. Retrieved 31 August 2016 from http://www.irrawaddy.com/burma/pan-ethnic-network-launches-promote-multilingual-education-burma.html.

Mod, Craig. 2016. "The Facebook-Loving Farmers of Myanmar." *The Atlantic,* 21 January. Retrieved 31 August 2016 from www.theatlantic.com/technology/archive/2016/01/thefacebooklovingfarmersofmyanmar/424812/.

Mookherji, Sangeeta, Garrett Mehl, Nadi Kaonga, and Patricia Mechael. 2015. "Unmet Need: Improving mHealth Evaluation Rigor to Build the Evidence Base." *Journal of Health Communication* 20(10): 1224–9.

Motlagh, Jason. 2014. "When a SIM Card Goes from $2,000 to $1.50." *Bloomberg,* 29 September. Retrieved 31 August 2016 from http://www.bloomberg.com/news/articles/2014-09-29/myanmar-opens-its-mobile-phone-market-cuing-carrier-frenzy.

"Myanmar: WHO Statistical Profile." 2013. WHO. Retrieved 31 August 2016 from http://www.who.int/gho/countries/mmr.pdf.

UN (United Nations). 2016. "Myanmar Country Profile." Retrieved 7 November 2017 from http://data.un.org/en/iso/mm.html.

Myat, Aye. 2014. "Ooredoo Launches Health App 'May May.'" *Myanmar Business Today,* 22 September. Retrieved 31 August 2016 from http://www.mmbiztoday.com/articles/ooredoo-launches-health-app-may-may.

Myers, Joe. 2016. "Which Are the World's Fastest-Growing Economies?" *World Economic Forum,* 18 April. Retrieved 31 August 2016 from https://www.weforum.org/agenda/2016/04/worlds-fastest-growing-economies/.

Salazar, N.B. 2010. "Towards an Anthropology of Cultural Mobilities." *Crossings: Journal of Migration and Culture* 1(1): 53–68.

Salazar, N.B., Elliot, A., & Norum, R. 2017. "Studying Mobilities: Theoretical Notes and Methodological Queries." In *Methodologies of Mobility: Ethnography and Experiment,* ed. A. Elliot, R. Norum, and N.B. Salazar, 1–24. Oxford: Berghahn Books.

Shealy, Shaina. 2016. "Providing Safe Illegal Abortions in Myanmar Is a 'Karmic Balance,' Says One Doctor." *PRI's The World,* 8 September. Retrieved 3 November 2016 from http://www.pri.org/stories/2016-09-08/providing-safe-illegal-abortions-myanmar-karmic-balance-says-one-doctor.

Trautwein, Catherine. 2014. "Ooredoo Delivers Maternity App." *Myanmar Times,* 22 September. Retrieved 31 August 2016 from http://www.mmtimes.com/index.php/business/technology/11744-ooredoo-delivers-maternity-app.html.

———. 2016. "Ooredoo Launches K30,000 Smartphone." *Myanmar Times,* 8 March. Retrieved 30 October 2016 from http://www.mmtimes.com/index.php/business/technology/19358-ooredoo-launches-k30-000-smartphone.html.

WHO (World Health Organization). 2011. *mHealth: New Horizons for Health through Mobile Technologies.* Global Observatory for eHealth series, Vol. 3. Geneva: WHO. Retrieved 1 December 2016 from http://www.who.int/goe/publications/goe_mhealth_web.pdf.

———. 2016. "New Checklist Published to Help Improve Reporting of mHealth Interventions." 22 March. Retrieved 31 August 2016 from http://www.who.int/reproductivehealth/topics/mhealth/mERA-checklist/en/.

World Bank. 2015. "Maternal Mortality Ratio (Modeled Estimate, per 100,000 Live Births)." Retrieved 31 August 2016 from http://data.worldbank.org/indicator/SH.STA.MMRT/countries/MM-TH-LA-KH-8S?display=graph.

———. 2016. "Literacy Rate, Adult Total (% of People Ages 15 and above)." Retrieved 7 November 2017 from http://data.worldbank.org/indicator/SE.ADT.LITR.ZS?locations=MM&year_high_desc=false.

Zainudeen, Ayesha, and Helani Galpaya. 2015. *Mobile Phones, Internet, and Gender in Myanmar.* Report of a joint GSMA Connected Women–LIRNEasia study. London: GSMA. Retrieved 31 August 2016 from http://www.gsma.com/mobilefordevelopment/wp-content/uploads/2016/02/GSMA_Myanmar_Gender_Web_Singles.pdf.

Postscript

Cecilia Vindrola-Padros, Ginger A. Johnson, and Anne E. Pfister

> Accounting for mobilities in the fullest sense challenges social science to change both the objects of its inquiries and the methodologies for research.
>
> —Kevin Hannam, Mimi Sheller, and John Urry, "Editorial: Mobilites, Immobilities and Moorings"

The chapters in this volume have sought to explore the ways in which healthcare is shaped by (im)mobilities and the different manifestations of (im)mobility forms as they occur in healthcare contexts. The case studies discussed in these chapters rise to the challenge put forth by Hannam et al. (2006) above, as the contributing authors have attempted to make sense of dynamic objects of inquiry in innovative ways.

Much has been written on the topics included in these chapters—on medical travel and tourism, healthcare worker migration, and mobile health. The purpose of this book is not to reproduce existing literature or rehash old arguments, but to make a case for the emergence of a new field of inquiry capable of encompassing all of these topics while posing new questions and theories. We argue that the use of mobility to obtain or deliver health services needs to be understood within a wider framework of healthcare (im)mobilities, in which we pay attention to both movement and stasis. In other words, this framework can capture the experiences of those who move and those who, as Castañeda proposed in her chapter, are "stuck in motion." This framework can examine health worker migration by capturing the experiences of workers who migrate, those who do not, and those who imagine or dream of migration (i.e., an imagined mobility that might never be enacted).

(Im)mobilities also need to be explored in processes of care delivery, whether through the use of strategies to reach isolated communities or through the establishment of aides to help patients navigate complex health systems or medical information (see Engelman, Edmiston, and Srinivas and Paphitis in this volume). These are all manifestations of the same area of inquiry, one that wishes to incorporate current theories and methods from the (im)mobilities literature into processes of healthcare access and delivery. In this brief closing chapter, we set out one proposal for how this might be achieved.

The Value of the Particular

The chapters in this volume have drawn from case studies in eight different regions of the world. These cross-cultural reflections on (im)mobilities in healthcare have pointed to some underlying themes uniting the experiences of patients, healthcare workers, and families at a global scale. One evident theme has been the important role played by contextual factors in shaping (im)mobility practices, experiences, and imaginaries. The authors have implemented a wide range of research approaches, but ethnographic research was predominantly used to capture the richness and particularities of the everyday (see, for instance, Kline, Speier, and Pfister and Vindrola-Padros in this volume).

These particularities of the everyday will need to be our focus in the field of healthcare (im)mobilities, as we need them to understand why and how each travel experience is different—why some can access healthcare easily, for example, while others struggle. This volume emphasizes the need to value these particularities as they provide insight into the wider processes that shape who (and what) moves, when they move, and how. Over twenty years ago, Lila Abu-Lughod (1991: 149) presented a critique of the concept of culture in anthropology and proposed instead that we develop "ethnographies of the particular." She argued that "by focusing closely on particular individuals and their changing relationships, one would necessarily subvert the most problematic connotations of culture: homogeneity, coherence, and timelessness" (p. 154). If we visualize (im)mobilities as components of these cultural practices, we can see how "ethnographies of the particular" can shed light on the heterogeneous, contradictory, and profoundly historical processes that affect our daily lives and our health.

Problematizing Healthcare (Im)mobilities

Through their analysis of particularities, the contributors to this volume have also pointed to evident inequalities in the use of mobility as a resource to guarantee healthcare access. The field of healthcare (im)mobilities will need to draw from critical perspectives to uncover how these inequalities are created and reproduced. This endeavor is particularly important in research carried out in healthcare contexts, as differential mobility empowerments might contribute to the distinction between those who can take action on behalf of their health and those who die avoidable deaths (see Čebron and Pistotnik in this volume).

As we consider the structures and processes that create populations understood as "deserving" and "undeserving" of healthcare, we must not lose sight of the ways in which individuals and systems are able to (re)configure these categories. "Ethnographies of the particular" provides a useful framework for understanding these categories, as this approach allows us to better capture the nuances of human actions, the (re)negotiation of power relations, and potential subversions of the social order. By working with and through health systems, and through movement that takes many forms, individuals take control of their healthcare-seeking behavior and the options available for the delivery of care. As the chapters in this collection demonstrate, when they are able to, people often go to great lengths to access high-quality care and, with appropriate resources, options often exist to provide services to distant populations.

(Im)mobilities as Theory and Method

The analysis of healthcare (im)mobilities sounds good in theory, but how can we advance this field from a methodological point of view? Several methods have been proposed in mobilities research to trace journeys, pathways, and flows of people, goods, and information (D'Andrea et al. 2011). Some have presented approaches whereby researchers become mobile, using "tracking methods," shadowing, or "walking along" techniques (Büscher and Urry 2009; Laurier et al. 2008; Spinney 2011). Another proposal is the use of multisited research and mobile ethnographies to document movement across both physical (i.e., fieldwork in multiple locales) and conceptual spaces (i.e., fieldwork covering various stages of a patient pathway) (Marcus 1995; Vergunst 2011). All of these approaches can be tried out in healthcare contexts, where researchers follow patients through journeys to obtain care (Speier 2017; Vindrola-Padros and Brage 2017), trace information flows involved in the use of technology in mHealth programs, or capture the multiple sites that healthcare workers inhabit while delivering care (see Plotnikova, and Briskin and Gallo in this volume).

An additional approach has been highlighted in another volume in this series (Elliot, Norum, and Salazar 2017), which entails the use of *immo-*

bility as a methodological approach. As Coates (2017: 112) has argued, "remaining immobile, still or strategically situated reveals much about the intersections between urban mobility and migrant experiences." By being "strategically situated," researchers are able to capture fluctuations in different ways. This might represent a novel approach in healthcare (im)mobilities, one we hope researchers will soon explore in more depth.

Concluding Thoughts

Healthcare in Motion emerged as a collaborative effort between scholars and practitioners to better understand mobilities and immobilities when accessing and delivering care. This volume incorporates new ways of conceptualizing movement and stasis in contexts of migration, social exclusion, deprivation, disease, discrimination, isolation, and (dis)ability. We believe this collection provokes interesting questions and provides methodological insight, and can serve as a starting point in the development of a new field of inquiry capable of understanding the complex healthcare problems our world faces—and the strategies we can use to address them.

Cecilia Vindrola-Padros, PhD, is a research associate in the Department of Applied Health Research, University College London, UK. She is a medical anthropologist and has researched the experiences of children and families who relocate to access medical treatment. Recent publications on mobility include the book chapters "Children Seeking Health Care: International Perspectives on Children's Use of Mobility to Obtain Health Services" (with Ginger Johnson), in *Mobilities and Journeys: Geographies of Children and Young People* (Springer, 2017), and "Child Medical Travel in Argentina: Narratives of Family Separation and Moving Away from Home" (with Eugenia Brage), in *Children's Health and Wellbeing in Urban Environments* (Routledge, 2017).

Ginger A. Johnson, PhD, is a visiting assistant professor at Southern Methodist University. She holds a PhD in medical anthropology and a master's degree in global public health from the University of South Florida and a master's degree in international law from the United Nations Interregional Crime and Justice Research Institute. Recently, she was embedded in West Africa conducting Ebola-related research with the International Federation of the Red Cross. A selection of her current research projects includes addressing adolescent nutritional needs in Cambodia, for the World Food Programme, and ensuring social accountability for maternal and child health in Malawi, for UNICEF.

Anne E. Pfister, PhD, is assistant professor of anthropology at the University of North Florida. Her research investigates how deaf youth and their families experience deafness in Mexico City by integrating sociocultural linguistic theory with biocultural medical anthropology analyses. Her project utilizes visual methods, including "photovoice," to actively engage participants as co-researchers. She has been involved with the Mexican deaf community for over ten years. Dr Pfister's research interests include disabilities studies, language socialization, and medicalization; her work has been published in *Ethos, Visual Anthropology Review, Behavioral and Brain Sciences, Collaborative Anthropologies,* and *Annals of Anthropological Practice.*

REFERENCES

Abu-Lughod, L. 1991. "Writing against Culture." In *Recapturing Anthropology: Working in the Present,* ed. R. G. Fox, 137–62. Santa Fe, NM: School of American Research Press.

Büscher, M., and J. Urry. 2009. "Mobile Methods and the Empirical." *European Journal of Social Theory* 12(1): 99–116.

Coates, J. 2017. "Idleness as Method: Hairdressers and Chinese Urban Mobility in Tokyo." In *Methodologies of Mobility: Ethnography and Experiment,* ed. A. Elliot, R. Norum, and N. B. Salazar, 109–28. New York: Berghahn Books.

D'Andrea, A., L. Ciolfi, and B. Gray. 2011. "Methodological Challenges and Innovations in Mobilities Research." *Mobilities* 6(2): 149–60.

Elliot, A., R. Norum, and N. B. Salazar, eds. 2017. *Methodologies of Mobility: Ethnography and Experiment.* New York: Berghahn Books.

Hannam, K., M. Sheller, and J. Urry. 2006. "Editorial: Mobilites, Immobilities and Moorings." *Mobilities* 1(1): 1–22.

Laurier, E., H. Lorimer, B. Brown, O. Jones, O. Juhlin, A. Noble, M. Perry, D. Pica, P. Sormani, I. Strebel, L. Swan, A. Taylor, L. Watts, and A. Weilenmann. (2008). "Driving and 'Passengering': Notes on the Ordinary Organization of Car Travel." *Mobilities* 3(1): 1–23.

Marcus G. 1995. "Ethnography in/of the World System: The Emergence of Multi-Sited Ethnography." *Annual Review of Anthropology* 24: 95–117.

Speier, A. 2017. *Fertility Holidays: IVF Tourism and the Reproduction of Whiteness.* New York: New York University Press.

Spinney, J. 2011. "A Chance to Catch a Breath: Using Mobile Video Ethnography in Cycling Research." *Mobilities* 6(2): 161–82.

Vergunst, J. 2011. "Technology and Technique in a Useful Ethnography of Movement." *Mobilities* 6(2): 203–19.

Vindrola-Padros, C., and E. Brage. 2017. "Child Medical Travel in Argentina: Narratives of Family Separation and Moving Away from Home." In *Children's Health and Wellbeing in Urban Environments,* ed. C. R. Ergler and R. A. Kearnes. London: Routledge.

Index

A
Abu-Lughod, Lila, 225
affective, 2
anthropology, 4, 225
asylum seekers, 54, 57, 61
Atlanta, Georgia, 4, 35–47
at-risk populations, 8, 149, 160
automobility, 4, 40–41, 48

B
barriers to care, 7–8, 48, 145, 165, 170–171, 177, 187, 190, 197, 216
bilingual, 91
biographical disruption, 82–83, 92
biographical reinforcement, 83
biographical work, 83
biomedical, 85–87, 90, 166, 192
Boal, Augusto, 152
bonding schemes, 124
borders, 1, 5, 13, 19, 30, 53, 57, 109–110, 117–119, 121, 128, 177–178
borderscapes, 30
brain circulation, 120
brain drain, 1, 118–119

C
capital, 3
caring, 4–5, 9, 74
caregiving, 84
carer, 2–3
children, 5–6, 22–26, 38–39, 43, 46, 59, 62, 74, 78–94, 100–101, 106–107, 109–111, 195, 213
citizen, 1,5, 20, 22–29, 59–60, 62–63, 123, 144, 159, 173, 203, 219
citizenship, 47, 57, 60, 66, 144, 158, 160
collaboration, 131, 156, 169, 179, 208, 217, 227
communication, 8, 143–147, 153–160, 168, 170–172, 179, 191–193, 202–205, 208–209, 216, 219
co-presence, 3
cross-border, 7, 20, 26, 100, 103–104, 112, 118–119, 121, 124–125, 129
culture, 27, 84, 91–92, 146, 155, 170–171, 191, 206–207, 216, 225
cure, 84, 86–87, 89
Czech Republic, 4, 6, 74, 99–112, 120

D
deserving, 4,9, 56, 62–63, 65, 226
deservingness, 1, 30, 40
destination, 7, 89, 93, 102, 104, 111, 120, 122–123, 126, 128–131
differential mobility empowerments, 4, 143, 226
disability, 74, 82–84, 87–88, 92–94, 143, 147–148, 195, 227
disadvantaged, 7, 22, 59, 66, 131
discourse, 30, 53, 56, 119, 126
discrimination, 7, 39, 56, 122, 160, 185–188
disparities, 7, 165, 187–189
displaced, 56
distance, 3, 28, 78, 140, 165, 191, 195, 197, 206
deaf, 6–8, 74, 77–93, 143–160
doctor, 24, 26, 28, 44–45, 58, 64, 86–88, 90, 100, 104, 108, 116–121, 131, 146, 155, 210–211

E
egg donation, 6, 99–100, 102–105, 107–112
emotion, 2, 40, 73, 79, 92–93, 193
empowerment, 56, 152, 156, 158–159, 226
ethics, 56, 61, 119, 122–123, 126–127, 129–130, 174, 176–177, 180
ethnography, 37, 80, 107
 ethnographies of the particular, 225–226

multisited ethnography, 37, 49
mobile ethnography, 49
erased, 5, 15, 54, 58, 60–66, 216
European Union, 57, 109, 117

F
family planning, 7, 9, 204
Feldman, A, 66
Freire, Paulo, 152

G
Garro, Linda, 74
gender, 2, 4, 7, 10, 36, 103, 160, 165, 185, 206–207
geographical constraints, 165
geographical mobility. *See* mobility
global economy, 112
globalization, 103
Grant, G., 82

H
hard-to-reach populations, 7, 139, 166, 168, 170, 179
HB2, 28, 186
HB 87, 38–39, 43
health
health coverage, 165
health inequalities, 4, 29
health insurance, 23–24, 27
health literacy, 58–61, 188
health promotion, 164, 166–171
health rights, 59–60
health workers, 3, 6–7, 48, 64–65, 116–131, 153, 158
healthcare
healthcare system, 2, 9, 16, 21, 55, 58–61, 63, 65, 110, 140, 167, 172, 178–179, 190, 192, 196–197
healthcare access, 3, 5, 7–10, 20–21, 23, 30, 37, 59, 141, 146, 186–187, 191, 194, 197, 225
healthcare landscape, 20, 192. *See also* landscape
hearing, 7–8, 78, 80–81, 84–88, 90, 92–93, 140, 144, 146–147, 149–150, 152, 154
HIV/AIDS, 7–9, 143–160, 166
HIV-positive, 8, 187, 194–195
history, 108, 188
horizontal scaling, 21

I
identity, 2, 6, 21, 23, 74, 80–84, 93–94, 104, 143, 186, 193, 195–197
illegality, 23, 39
imaginaries, 6–7, 74–75, 93, 100, 112, 225
imagination, 6, 16, 73–75, 83, 110–111
immigration policies, 4, 128
immigration policing, 38
immobility, 5, 15–16, 20, 30, 41, 61, 144, 151, 153, 157, 159, 215
infertility, 100–101, 103–104
informal providers, 29, 42, 47
interviews, 21, 37, 90, 101, 105, 144–145
intimate labor, 105, 109
in vitro fertilization, 101
IPPLIAP, 77–80, 85, 90, 92–93

J
Journey, 2, 6–7, 24, 25, 78, 80–81, 84, 86–87, 89, 93, 103, 120, 226

K
Kangas, Beth, 3
Kenya, 4, 7–8, 140, 143–160
Kenyan Sign Language (KSL), 8, 146, 148, 150
Khan, Nichola, 5

L
landscape, 2, 9, 19–20, 40, 192, 203, 215
language, 8, 22, 53, 78–80, 84–86, 90–91, 94, 121–123, 128, 146–148, 151, 154–155, 157, 168, 171–172, 205, 211, 215–216, 218
LGBT, 186–190, 198
liminality, 5, 15, 66
LVCT Health, 8, 144–145, 147–149, 151, 153, 155–160

M
maldistribution, 116, 165
marginalized, 7, 64, 66, 140, 143, 156, 158, 178, 188
maymay, 9, 203, 207–220
meaning, 2, 3, 5, 19, 74, 79, 83, 91–92, 100, 112, 154, 165, 168, 177, 207
Medicaid, 22–26, 29, 194
medical travel, 224
medical tourism, 3, 100, 103

medications, 26–29, 99, 101, 110, 154, 167, 169, 171, 173–174, 177, 193
medication literacy, 167
medicine information leaflets (MILs), 172–174, 176–177, 179
Mexico, 4, 20–30, 41, 45, 90–91
Mexico City, 6, 74, 77–80, 84–87, 89
mhealth, 1, 7–8, 140, 144, 158–159, 214–217, 219, 226
mHealth evidence and reporting assessment (mERA) checklist, 214–215
minority, 91, 143, 156, 160, 188
Mobile Alliance for Maternal Action (MAMA), 208, 210–211, 217
mobile clinics, 8, 168
mobile ethnographic methods, 16
mobile phones, 158, 205–207, 215, 219
mobile technology, 158–159, 215
mobilities turn, 144
mobility
  cross-border mobility, 118–119, 129, 131
  cultural mobility, 6, 100, 111–112
  economic mobility, 40, 107, 112
  geographical mobility, 118, 166
  health-related, 36, 41, 43, 48
  micro-mobility, 100, 192, 197
  limited mobility, 9, 36, 47, 187, 197
  physical mobility, 9, 73, 165
  regulation of mobility, 19, 21, 65
moorings, 5, 224
motility, 5–6
motion, 5–6, 20, 30, 73, 80, 177–178, 224
movement, 1–10, 15–16, 19–20, 30, 36, 39–40, 47, 73–75, 81, 84, 88, 92–94, 100, 112, 120–125, 139, 158, 165–168, 178, 185, 192–193, 196, 215, 224, 226–227
multisited ethnography. *See* ethnography
Myanmar, 4, 7, 9, 140, 202–219

N
Nairobi, 145, 147–149, 151, 157–159
Nashville, Tennessee, 9, 190
narrative, 6, 74–75, 80–84, 86–89, 93–94
navigation, 4, 7, 88, 167, 216
network, 3, 9, 89, 121, 129, 151, 153, 158, 165, 189, 204–205, 214, 216
noncitizen, 57, 60, 62
non-governmental organization (NGO), 8, 37, 129–130, 144, 147, 155–156, 158, 202, 214
nurses, 42, 99, 101, 106, 116–121, 126–128, 155, 165, 169, 195

P
parents, 6, 24–25, 28–29, 39, 46, 74, 80–81, 83–94, 100–106, 111–112, 195
participant observation, 21, 101, 105, 145
participatory theater, 8, 151–152
pathology, 87
patient, 1–4, 7–9, 27, 29, 42–43, 46–47, 54, 58, 63, 89, 99–100, 102, 104–107, 109, 110, 121–124, 140, 165–173, 177–179, 187, 190–197, 214, 224–226
pharmacy, 4, 8, 168, 170–176, 178–179
Phelophepa Healthcare Trains, 167–171, 173–174, 177–179
place, 1–5, 20, 29, 30, 37–38, 42, 47–49, 54, 57, 73, 82, 89, 103, 144, 151, 177–178, 193, 208
poaching, 121
policing, 22, 27, 44–45. *See also* immigrant policing
policy, 4, 6–7, 20–21, 30, 39, 48–49, 118–119, 123–124, 126, 127–131, 139, 148, 156–157, 172, 188, 190
post-social state, 56–57, 62, 65–66
potential, 3, 5–8, 38–39, 42, 64, 81–82, 84, 104, 108, 111, 130, 144–145, 157–160, 167, 193–194, 215, 217, 226
Prague, 99–101, 109–112
PSI-M, 202–204, 207–212, 214, 216–219

Q
qualitative research, 189

R
recruitment, 100, 104, 119, 121–123, 125, 127–131
refugees, 53–54, 58
representation, 122, 168
reproduction, 102–103
reproductive medicine, 99, 101–102, 104
resistance, 90, 108
rural, 7–8, 24, 40, 120, 122, 140, 145, 147, 151, 153–154, 157–159,

164–168, 170, 172, 179, 187–189, 191, 194, 197, 204–206, 216, 218

S

Salazar, Noel, 112, 144, 206, 215
Slovenia, 4–5, 15, 53–55, 57–62, 64–69
self-deport, 39, 47, 49
service learning, 8, 140, 173–175, 178
sickness, 211
socialist state, 55
South Africa, 4, 8, 120, 126, 140, 153, 165–173, 176–179, 208
space, 2, 5, 9, 16, 21, 37–38, 40–42, 46–47, 49, 66, 90–91, 93–94, 101, 155, 159, 166–167, 178, 186, 189, 192, 196–197, 207, 218–219, 226
stasis, 2, 3, 5, 10, 15, 36, 140, 167, 224, 227
story, 25–26, 44, 82–84, 88, 108, 155
stuck in motion, 5, 20, 30, 224
stuckness, 5, 15, 30, 61
students, 8, 59, 77, 85, 106, 108, 110, 118, 127, 152, 167, 169–171, 173–177, 195
subjective, 3

T

technology, 3, 87, 139–141, 143–145, 158–160, 173, 179, 202–203, 205, 207–208, 214–216, 219, 226
Tesfahuney, M, 4
Texas, 4, 20, 22, 28
transgender, 8–9, 140, 185–197
Trans Buddy Program, 9, 190–191, 194–197
time, 9, 16, 20, 24, 27, 29, 41, 43, 45, 56, 65, 77, 80–85, 87–93, 100, 106–107, 110, 112, 117, 144, 158, 165, 170, 178, 190, 193, 203, 208, 214–215
tourism, 3, 6, 100, 102–103, 224. *See also* medical tourism
transportation, 24, 28, 40, 42, 46, 48, 77, 85, 119, 153, 186, 188, 191, 194
travel, 3, 5–6, 19, 20, 22, 25–30, 53, 74, 78–93, 99, 102–112, 119, 122, 151, 165, 168, 186–187, 190–191, 195–197, 225–226
  corporeal travel, 6
  imagined travel, 6, 75
  performed travel, 6

U

undeserving, 5, 39–40, 48, 56, 58, 61–63, 65–66, 226
undocumented, 4–5, 15–16, 20–29, 35–49, 54, 57, 61
United States, 4, 5, 15, 20–30, 38–40, 43, 47–48, 102, 103, 106, 108–109, 111, 117, 120, 155, 186–188, 215
urgent treatment, 58, 63

V

vertical scaling, 21
visa, 22, 27
Voluntary Counseling and Testing (VCT), 8, 144–160
vulnerable, 7, 16, 48–49, 63, 65, 117, 140, 147, 156, 165

W

waiting, 15–16, 101–102, 152, 186, 190, 193, 205
Wilson, S., 83
workforce, 62, 64, 75, 109, 116–119, 123, 125–126, 130–131

Y

Yugoslavia, 57–58

www.ingramcontent.com/pod-product-compliance
Ingram Content Group UK Ltd.
Pitfield, Milton Keynes, MK11 3LW, UK
UKHW021837100926
8556IPUK00004B/399

9 781785 339530